Weight Loss Is Not Wellness

Taking you to new heights of human potential through Super Health, Super Money, Fat Burning-Weight Loss, and Incredible Love

LIVE SUPERHUMAN

By
Dr. Rook Torres

For Shade and Kyen

The soul of my inspiration,
I love you 100 percent...no matter what.
May your life be filled with unimaginable good.

Indescribable thanks to:
Dad, Mom, Simi, and Troy, for displaying the **actions** of unconditional love, friendship, and support that most can't put into **words**.

My darling wife Helen for always looking out for me—and helping me master myself.

Additional thanks to Rachael Daigle
for her astute, watchful eye and guidance.

Weight Loss Is Not Wellness
Your Breakthrough Guide for Living a Super Human Lifestyle Without Dieting

Sabre Enterprises, LLC
8314 W. Pamela St.
Boise, ID 83714
www.sabre-ebooks.com

ISBN: 978-0615549798 (Printed Version)
978-1450783996 (Electronic Version)

Printed in the United States of America on post-consumer recycled paper

Sabre-eBooks.com

Table of contents:

Section 1		page
Chapter 1	Could This Be Me?	1
Chapter 2	Weight Loss Is NOT Wellness	3
Chapter 3	The SuperHuman Code	5
Section 2	**The 5 Blessings**	
Chapter 4	The 5 Blessings	15
Chapter 5	The Blessing of Safety	19
Chapter 6	The Blessing of Love	23
Chapter 7	The Blessing of Health	29
Chapter 8	The Blessing of Happiness	33
Chapter 9	The Blessing of Prosperity	39
Section 3	**SuperHuman Elements of Wellness**	
Chapter 10	The 3 SuperHuman Elements of Wellness	45
Chapter 11	Physical Element: Strength	47
Chapter 12	Flexibility, Movement, and Alignment	51
Chapter 13	SuperHuman Elements of Wellness: BioChemical	57
Chapter 14	Creating Wellness Not Just Weight Loss	59
Chapter 15	How Do I Eat?	69
Chapter 16	Do SuperHumans Take Nutritional Supplements?	73
Chapter 17	GAP	77
Section 3.1	**Bio-Chemical Myths...Busted!**	
Chapter 18	Drinking Milk Can Make You Fat	81
Chapter 19	A New Cure for Cancer: Theory or Reality?	87
Chapter 20	Bad Medicine	93
Chapter 21	Why Can Drugs Be So Bad?	97
Chapter 22	Heart Attacks and Cholesterol	101
Chapter 23	Bad Supplements Can Kill You	109
Chapter 24	Never Sick...No Problem	115
Chapter 25	Injecting Poison	119
Chapter 26	Childhood Vaccinations: Blind Shots	123
Chapter 27	SuperHuman Elements of Wellness: Neuro-Spiritual	127
Section 4		
Chapter 28	Purpose	133
Chapter 29	Selflessness	137
Chapter 30	Passion to Prosperity	141
Chapter 31	Cleaning House	151
Chapter 32	You Matter	153
Live SuperHuman Tool Summary		155

Introduction

Live truth instead of professing it. –Elbert Hubbard

I am not a guy who goes out every morning at 5:00 a.m. and runs five miles with my family. I'm not a vegetarian or raw foodist, and I don't eat all organic food all of the time. I don't work out for hours on end and torture myself in the gym. I'm not happy 100 percent of the time, and I do have stress. I'm also not a guy who tells people to do these things to live well. I don't represent a tiny percentage of people who live in a way that few others can duplicate. I was once told by a patient that he came to see me even though he wouldn't normally consider seeing a chiropractor because he could sense I live in a way that represents wellness. He could tell when he met me that wellness was coming out of me. "It was who you are," he said. Then he said he's not a guy who does all that stuff listed above either but he thought he could learn from my example. What he meant is that I am a real, down to earth practioner of wellness, not some phony faker selling him a scheme he could never duplicate.

So what do I do? I do work out an average of three to four times a week. Often, I get up early to play basketball and lift weights, but I make sure I enjoy it. I never torture myself. I have healthy protein shakes for breakfast sometimes but I also love homemade egg sandwiches. I eat red meat a few times a month, and chips and chocolate are my favorite less healthy snacks. However, I do strive to eat healthy a majority of the time, following the guidelines I recommend in this book.

Do I have charisma for life and a positive outlook, absolutely! I live what I talk about in this book, not more not less. I am determined to send the message you'll read about in this book, which is why I've worked so hard to be a good example. I know that deep down most of us feel like we could achieve more. I know, for sure, that you can apply the principles and tools in this book, and you will become more than you currently are. I know because I have done it.

Simple. That's how I want you to think about your life and health starting now. In this book you will learn about the Wellness Spectrum (chapter 27 and 32) and you will determine where on that spectrum you are and where you want to be. I will personally teach you simple, small steps and changes to improve your state of being. If you finish this book and then try to implement every suggestion at once you will fail. The process is not about achieving health and wellness tomorrow. It is about implementing consistent, small changes over time so that in one month, six months, one year, even ten years from now, you are healthier than you are today. By implementing the countless lessons in this book and at my website **www.LiveSuperHuman.com**, you make the small changes that will lead you to your own success.

People have said to me: "You're so lucky to be so healthy." But I can assure you that health has little to do with luck and everything to do with choices. All you have to do is start making the right choices.

I do not want to motivate you!

Motivate, as in "an incentive for action; to move," is a classic outside-in technique for managing others. Motivation is like a drug that only temporarily changes you. Stop taking the drug and the symptoms return. Instead of motivation.

...I want to inspire you!

Inspire, as I define it, is "a spiritual breath into." Motivate is something you do. Inspire is something you are. It begins by being the change you want to see in the world, to show up in such a way that people think, "I would like to be like him/her."

Be inspirational, and not only will we have the opportunity to change lives, we'll change the world.

Section 1

Chapter 1

Could This Be Me?

I walk into the room like I've done literally thousands of times before, never knowing what to expect. Within seconds I get used to the slight stinging, sulfuric smell of developing chemicals seeping under the door to the dark room. The exam room is very small—only eight by eight feet—but sort of comfortable, just how I designed it, knowing that would keep the amount of time spent in here to a minimum. Not this time.

Waiting for me is a woman barely 30 years old with beautiful skin and a charming smile. But deep behind her eyes is a profound hurt, which is almost undetectable behind a veil built by years of self preservation and strength. My heart sinks. She has a gleaming personality that immediately makes it hard to notice she is drastically overweight, perhaps by more than 200 pounds. I begin to think to myself how much I can never understand what is must be like to be her.

After a typical brief consultation about her complaints related to a car accident and an explanation as to how I can help, the real doctor in me begins to get brave enough to be dead honest with her. As sensitive as I can be, I softly say, "I need to speak honestly so, tell me, if you don't mind, about your weight. Are you happy with it or is it a goal to change it?" Immediately, as if she needed to vent, she tells me how badly she wants to lose weight but no matter what she does it won't happen for her and that it's been like that her whole life. She explains how she has read many books and rattles off more information about experts in the "diet" world than even I know. She explains, while starting to cry, what it is like to be judged by people who think she eats junk food all the time and how she works out for two hours nearly every day with almost no success in losing weight.

My heart breaks and I struggle to fight back some pressing tears. I think to myself what it must be like to be a girl who has grown trying to feel beautiful her whole life, has done a better job than most people at doing so, yet never can feel fulfilled. What it is like to always be on the search for the next thing that may help you feel whole and accepted and above all else, free from your own prison.

Man or woman, overweight or not, I think we all have a powerful desire to feel whole, accepted and free. I'll even go as far as to say feeling this way is your right given to you by your Source, or God, at birth and then somehow partially or completely lost by some of us. The search to regain this right consumes many people's entire lives and others never seem to have lost it at all. This book will help anyone who is in the game, searching for or craving more complete wholeness or a higher degree of wellness. I will inspire you with what I call the 5 Blessings, to help you reclaim natural and true wellness. If you think you just need to lose weight to solve your problems, that in itself is a sign of a deeper problem. That is why I say "weight loss is NOT wellness."

The beautiful woman described earlier is the perfect example of someone who could apply the tools in this book and start making change for the better right now. Unfortunately, I only got the chance to work with her for a few short months. In that time her constant, severe pain, which had kept her from working out, completely resolved. She felt bad for not being more active and by helping her heal herself, she was then able to feel better about herself and become more active as well.

You don't have to be in the dire situation this woman felt she was in to benefit from the Live SuperHuman principles. In fact, I know that wherever you are on your own path in life, this book will help take you to where you want to go!

Chapter 2

Weight Loss Is NOT Wellness

"What do you mean weight loss is not wellness? If I lose weight won't I be healthy? Are you telling me that I won't be? Everyone says to lose weight, my doctor, my mom or dad, my wife or husband, books and "experts." If I lose the extra 10, 20, 50, 100, or more pounds that I've been carrying, won't that give me more wellness?"

The most honest answer I can give you to these questions is this: Yes, you will be able to achieve more wellness if you lose excess weight. However, getting to, or close to, your ideal weight does not mean you will be healthy or have an ideal level of wellness. Remember, weight is one small part of wellness and many people who are at their ideal weight are far from healthy. So, if you lose "the weight" will you be healthy? Not necessarily. This is the difference between being human and living SuperHuman.

Together, we are going to take a journey to a new place. Not a simple lateral shift or an experience that feels good but doesn't really take you anywhere, like sitting in a hot tub. I'm talking about a transformation, like discovering an entirely new set of abilities you never even knew you had. I'm talking about developing some of the skills and abilities that you may know you have or may be unknown to you completely, into skills and abilities that are so strong you will barely recognize your old self. I'm talking about developing a new code to live by, the new way to eat and nourish your body, a new way to think about yourself in relation to others, and a new way to physically shape your body. Get ready to learn the secrets that many people have learned and implemented in their lives that have taken them to great heights. Get ready to Live SuperHuman.

Throughout the book you will find pages like this specifically designed for you to take notes, record thoughts, or highlight something special that you have learned. Super helpful...we think so too...you're welcome!

Chapter 3

The SuperHuman Code

The Live SuperHuman code is made up of 14 core values that SuperHumans live by. These core values help you develop and strengthen the super powers you have. By super powers, I don't mean mythical powers, but rather, real powers that if developed, drive human beings to rise up to living life to a higher standard. A standard that lifts all of those around them through example, literally not figuratively. This is your *personal* code.

The Live SuperHuman code:

1. always maximize your powers, never give them up
2. always share your powers with as many people as possible
3. always help others and the world whenever you can
4. always use your superpowers to save lives
5. never doubt
6. never fear
7. never underestimate the power of positive thinking
8. always be honest with yourself
9. always be authentic
10. always be safe
11. always love the moment
12. always live healthy
13. always share your happiness with others
14. always know everything grows and prospers and so do you!

One thing you notice when you read the code above is that they are all absolutes beginning with "always" and "never." I don't want to be unrealistic with regard to the nature of our lives and I understand that it is near impossible to do anything 100 percent of the time. You could argue that fear, for example, is necessary in some situations. I agree, however, I will say that fear is used mostly in life as a mechanism to keep you safe. Thus, code number 10, always be safe has you covered. Remember that this is your personal code for you, and all about you moving forward in life. So think of number five, never doubt, as it applies to you specifically as in never doubt yourself or your self-confidence.

Have you ever wanted to have super powers? What powers would you choose? Flying? Invincibility? Laser vision? Super strength? Invisibility? Super speed? Mind reading? At one point or another everyone has been asked this question or at least thought about it. The truth is, most of us would love to have any one of the super powers rather than just dream about what it would be like. Instead, most people settle for believing they don't have even one.

Believing you do not have any super powers is a sad thought. I have come to believe that we all have super powers! What is even sadder is that we don't call them, or think of them, as super powers at all. "What do you mean, I have super powers?" You ask. I'm glad to answer that question and, as a matter of fact, I'm going to lead you on a journey in the upcoming pages that will make you feel so powerful that you will become SuperHuman, not just believe you are. You are going to feel so powerful that not only will you want to take your new powers and put them to use for yourself right away, you will have the ability to use them for the good of others as well! You will become so abundantly powerful that I'm going to show you how, together, we can change the world in a very short period of time by sharing the gifts of our powers with others! This is not an empty claim. This, my friend, is my guarantee to you. Read on and so that you can begin to Live SuperHuman.

I would like to share with you the secrets that I am so grateful to have learned and been able to share with my patients over the past decade. In my current practice, which spans one third of my life, I have cared for over 4000 different cases and well over 100,000 office visits, consultations, and interviews. I use the best, most advanced technology available on the planet for my profession to analyze and monitor people's results. I have also personally reviewed over 4,000 published articles from various sources like medical journals and trade publications. I have cared for many professional athletes and a few celebrities. You may think "Wow, thousands of office visits, that's a lot!" and it is, compared to some, which gives me powerful knowledge to share with you. However, I must also acknowledge all my incredible colleagues in chiropractic who have seen many, many more patients than I have. It is not only great for me to honor each Doctor of Chiropractic in this book but it is also terrific news for you because one of these incredible doctors is probably located near you just waiting for you to contact them so they can share this knowledge with you and help you with the programs I have designed here.

The point is, the programs, tips and recommendations I have put together for you will undoubtedly help you find freedom from the suffering you are going through, whether it's sickness, disease, financial stress, physical pain, negativity, or relationship problems. These are most people's daily stresses and they are issues that you will learn to process out or decrease as you begin to Live SuperHuman.

As a person who is about to experience the ability to identify and develop super powers I want you recognize, that first, you will need your new code to live by. This code that will give you a foundation and the fundamentals for your new thoughts, actions and behaviors. The code will not necessarily give you a purpose (we will cover that also) but it will give you rules to help manage and utilize your new abilities to your full potential. Think of yourself as a bird teaching another bird how to fly. You can't just say "flap your wings and good luck." You would have to explain how the way you flap your wings, the angle, the breadth, the tilt, drag, wind, air pockets, gusts, risers, temperature, moisture, tail function, and so on will determine the power or your flight. Then you lead by example. This is how you get yourself and others to a more powerful place. It takes help from those who have gone before and made contact with the next level. The Live Superhuman code will help you get there. And it is part of our journey to help one another get there.

Charging Your Super Powers Everyday

I realize that not everyone wants to achieve the same thing with their health but naturally we all want more wellness in life because life is just better when you are strong and healthy. That is the beauty of getting what you want. Everyone can get what they want because we don't all want the same things. Even the things we all do want are so abundant they can't be depleted. Impossible you might think but what about air? Not only do we all want air, we need it! The average person takes around 21,600 breathes in a 24 hour period. That means some people take double that and some people take less than that. Can you imagine telling the person next to you, "hey pal, would you mind not breathing so much, you're hogging the air!?" They can have as much as they want and you know there will be enough for you and everyone else on the planet, including the animals, plants, fires, chemical reactions, and so on, that need it.

This is the beauty of the abundance of the universe we live in, it is literally as big as you can imagine. I also believe that things exist in this way to teach us about ourselves, so pay attention. So let's start thinking bigger and expand ourselves so that our possibilities expand as well.

Live SuperHuman Tool: **Thinking bigger and more creatively is a way to charge up and become more powerful.**

How to Start Your Day

Typically I wake up early to prepare for my day (I love to sleep in and I believe you should now and then). The very first thing that I do is say or think "thank you, thank you so much." Who am I thanking? I'm thanking my Source, God (or GOD 'the Grand Organized Design' if you prefer), the air I breathe in, my wife for keeping me warm. If my son has climbed into bed with me in the morning, I thank him. I thank the endless energy and love I have. I thank my guardian angels. I thank anything and everything that makes me thankful. The idea is to fill yourself with gratitude.

One of my favorite teachers and speakers is healer and philosopher Dr. John Demartini. He speaks about love and gratitude as being foundational to having the life of your dreams, and he's right. Through all the reading and searching I have done, I have found that being thankful is the best place to start not only your day, but it's also the best place to start building a foundation for who you are. If you have gratitude, oozing out of you, you can use that to begin driving things you want toward you at light speed! Think about it: isn't being grateful for what you have one of the best ways to humble yourself and get more of the things you want. If you gave someone a gift and they were ungrateful, would that make you feel good? Would it make you want to give them another gift? No way! But if you gave a gift to someone and they genuinely thanked you, and you could literally feel how good they feel because they expressed so much gratitude, you would be glad to give to them again. It would likely encourage you to give to others as well. You may even feel so good from their gratitude that you feel like you got the gift. Actually, you did. You gave yourself a gift through them and that is why giving feels so good.

Gratitude is powerful. Dr. Demartini says he does not get out of bed in the morning until he gets a tear of gratitude in his eye. I don't cry much, but if I do it is usually "tears of happiness," because I'm so thankful or happy to be in that moment witnessing whatever it is. Experience this regularly. No matter where you are, physically or metaphorically, gratitude can be with you.

Each morning, as I head to the bathroom to brush my teeth after climbing out of bed I start to feel more powerful because of the energy of gratitude.

Live SuperHuman Tool: **Gratitude builds your power.**

The next thing I do is yoga. Yoga is a way to create an experience for yourself and a great way to live in the moment. I tell all my patients "yoga is like brushing your teeth for your spine." I love yoga in the morning to loosen up my body, help me feel strong, flexible and powerful. I have developed a short yoga routine that is perfect for me and I've shared with you at LiveSuperHuman.com so you can make it your own if you choose. There are so many options to take advantage of when it comes to learning yoga. Your local gym, YMCA, or yoga studios are all great places to get more instruction. This graceful routine takes me about 10 minutes and charges me for the day. It invigorates my soul and deepens my sense of connection with myself and the world as I get to experience my body doing something beautiful for the first time that day. I breathe deeply and slowly, feeling my muscles loosen, loving the feeling of each pose. Yoga prepares my mind and my body as I transition my yoga routine into the next step, meditation.

Live SuperHuman Tool: **Yoga will make you physically and Neuro-Spiritually more powerful.**

Meditation is so simple, but do not confuse it with other types of difficult meditation you have heard of. There are many different types of meditation developed by different cultures or for specific purposes. What is important for you to learn is what is effective for you. I have tried different types of meditation and found that I like nearly all of them. However, some are much easier than others. What works best for me is two specific ways to meditate. The first meditation I do is morning meditation. This meditation is discussed in detail. It is the primary focus of this book, and it is how I received the idea to write this book. The morning meditation is The 5 Blessings which are explained in detail in section two.

One of my favorite quotes is from Dr. Wayne Dyer, whom I have met and have great admiration for. I've heard him say, "if prayer is you talking to God, then intuition is God talking to you." This is one of the main reasons I meditate differently at night and in the morning. My morning meditation is an active meditation that stimulates my mind and gives me many ideas. My nighttime meditation is more peaceful and quiets my mind.

The second meditation is a nighttime routine that I have found works better for me because it calms my mind for healing and receiving insight during sleep. In my nighttime meditation I simply set a timer for whatever amount of time feels good at the moment. Usually seven minutes is the shortest amount of time and twenty minutes is the longest. I simply sit next to my wife in bed with pillows behind our backs up against our headboard. I dim the lights and set my timer, which plays beautiful, gentle harp music when the time is up. Then I close my eyes and simply focus on my breathing. Breathe in…breathe out…in…out. When a thought pops into my head, I simply return my focus to my breathing and try not to get too carried away in the thought. Sometimes you will find one thought leads to another, which leads to another until you have a whole story going on in your head. If this happens, and you get carried away, gently return your focus to your breathing. As you do more and more meditation you will find it easier and easier to keep your focus and fewer thoughts will appear. Know in advance that thoughts pop into your head all the time and you really have little control at first. Simply return your focus to your breathing and do not be agitated by your thoughts.

Another thing I like to do before I meditate is set an intention that my subconscious mind can work on attracting while my conscious mind is resting. For example, something I intend to attract into my life is new people I can help. Or perhaps I would like to attract more money that week, or heal an injury. Maybe I intend to have a new idea for a product or book. Whatever the intention is, I simply state it or write it down and then begin relaxing my mind.

Live SuperHuman Tool: **Meditate to increase wellness, Physically and Neuro-Spiritually.**

This is an easy first step you can do starting now, and I suggest you start tonight. You will sleep better, wake up more energized, have clearer thinking and more focus the next day. You will notice new ideas come easier and your ability to act on them is more natural to you. All of these things will benefit you. Start tonight; there is no reason to delay! You don't need to be spiritual or religious. Meditation has nothing to do with either. This practice has to do with you and your life and your connection to the universe you live in, not outside influences or beliefs.

One last tip I'd like to offer is about larger intentions—like resolutions or big goals. If you like to make a New Year's resolution every year or set big goals that you intend to achieve at some point in the future, then I would like to share a story with you. This story is about making sure you are specific with your targets when you set your goals. One year, as I was still really learning the SuperHuman Code, I decided to make a New Year's resolution. I had never actually made one before because I thought it was something people did when they didn't have the ability to focus on achieving what they want. I also considered New Year's resolutions to be big things, not small things like losing a pound or two or to stop eating peanut butter for a week. Of course, the truth is that a resolution or a goal can be what ever you want to be, big or small. Anyway, for the first time I decided that I wanted to set a New Year's resolution and this one I thought was the perfect resolution: I was going to get out of debt that year. I thought it was a perfect goal and although I didn't know how it was going to happen, I set my intention and I let it go, knowing that magically at the end of the year I would have achieved what I set out to achieve.

Well, to make a long story short, after some investments went bad, I wound up having to decide whether or not I would file for bankruptcy or sell my business to wipe out my debt. When I started the year with a vision of being debt-free those options were not exactly what I had in mind. So please, learn from my mistake and when you set a goal or a resolution and you write it down be sure that you also outline the path you'd like to take to get there. Of course, it wasn't the end of the world for me and down the line things worked out very well. I was even able to write this book to help you learn from me.

In the upcoming chapters, you'll read what inspired me to write this book. The fundamentals to begin to Live SuperHuman are outlined for you in great detail. Utilize all these tools on a daily basis to help make your world and the world of others a better place.

Section 2

Chapter 4

The 5 Blessings

It became very clear to me in a relatively short period of time that I had to share the 5 Blessings with as many people as possible. My goal became to share with others how I bring the 5 Blessings into my life so that others may know them, too. The process is based on thousands of years of spiritual practices, cutting edge neuro science, and very current and advanced research studies that validate this amazing process. In short, this is what I meditate on: I imagine that everyone I know, no matter where they are, is given 5 blessings. These blessings are 5 force fields, or protective bubbles, that surround each of them at all times. Those blessings are:

Safety: I wish them blessed with ultimate protection from harm.
Love: I wish them abundantly blessed with the greatest power ever known.
Health: I wish them spectacular physical and mental health.
Happiness: I wish them laughter, smiles and deep internal bliss throughout life.
Prosperity: I wish them the lifestyle they dream of.

If we each swirled these thoughts around in our heads all of the time, or even once a day, how do you think our world would be? If we were to actually focus these thoughts toward others, how do you think things around you might change? I think we all know it would be different for sure. When I offer these blessings to every person I know, and you offer them to everyone you know, and so on, we can cover the globe with a powerful positive message and energy in a very short amount of time.

Studies show that the average person knows approximately 65 people they could call on the phone and have a conversation with. Some know less and some many more, but let's say you offer the blessings to 65 people, those 65 each offer the blessings to 65, those 65 to 65 each, and those 65 each offer the blessings to 65 more and it happens one more time. Get ready because this is truly SuperHuman! That is 65 to the 5th power, and we will be spreading safety, love, health, happiness, and prosperity to over 1.1 billion people world wide! If it spreads just a little bit more, this incredible energy will reach every living thing on earth! We will all be giving great amounts of good from our hearts to everything and everyone we care about every single day. This is the essence of saving the world. It is the essence of being a super hero, the essence of being SuperHuman!

You might ask, "Who am I to give out blessings?" And the answer is, "you are a part of the energy that makes up this universe. If you take a powerful microscope and zoom in close enough on any substance, you see the smallest particles like protons and neutrons and subatomic particles like leptons, photons and bosons. Beyond that, there are no more particles; there is just energy. In terms of God, it is God's universe, and you are a very real part of it. Whatever terminology you prefer when it comes to God or energy is up to you. Remember, energy can never be created or destroyed, it only changes form. Trees bless us with shade, beauty and oxygen. The sun blesses us with energy, warmth and light. Animals bless us with love, clothing and food. You have every right to offer helpful blessings just as anyone or anything else on the planet. Our personal, preferably positive, energy is one of the most powerful forms of energy on the planet, and it is not only within our ability to send out positive energy, which I choose to call a blessing, but I feel that it is our ethical responsibility. It is an obligation of a SuperHuman.

Live SuperHuman Tool: **Share positive energy with everyone you know in the form of a blessing. You never know who may need it right now.**

Before you think this is a kooky pipe dream without scientific basis or the possibility to be proven, I'd like you to consider the following triple blind study done by one of the greatest researchers—and definite SuperHumans—of our time. Dr. Masaru Emoto has become world-famous by studying energetic intention on water. Dr. Emoto developed a process to flash freeze water after it has been subjected to various positive or negative stimuli. He then analyzes the crystals formed by the frozen water. In a recent study 1,900 people in Austria and Germany were instructed to focus positive intention, over three days, toward water sealed in an electromagnetically shielded room in Los Angeles, California. Other water samples were placed right next to the study water, but unknown to the test subjects sending positive intention. Both water samples were placed inside the same shielded room. Drops taken from both samples of water in the different treatment conditions (one zapped with positivity and the other not zapped) were frozen and photographed by a technician. The photographs were analyzed and rated for aesthetic beauty by 2,500 independent judges. The results of the crystal images from the treated condition or "zapped", were rated as aesthetically more beautiful by the judges a majority of the time (1).

Not only is the study remarkable because it measures people's positive energy, but it measures positive energy sent over nearly 6,000 miles. On top of that, the energy penetrated an energy-shielded room. What makes the study even more amazing is the fact that it was a triple blind study, which means that the people sending positive intention to the water didn't know there were two water samples. And the people rating the photographs of the frozen water samples didn't know which was which. This study absolutely blows my mind and opens possibilities for people that I only have dreamed about!

The logical next question is: Can one person affect another person's safety, love, health, happiness or prosperity from a distance by simply thinking about it or intending it to happen? I wager that it can be done. Because I, like everyone, have been in situations where I have walked into a room where two people are having a disagreement and physically been able to feel the negative energy. On the other hand, I have been around people who are happy and enthusiastic and can feel very real good energy. Everyone has had a similar experience in one way or another; it's time to use that knowledge and those experiences for the benefit of others.

In the coming chapters you'll discover how to harness your NeuroSpiritual SuperHuman tools to send blessings and intentions to yourself and others, just as I do. I personally invite you make the 5 Blessings your daily meditation and add these "weapons of good" to your arsenal. Imagine you are a super hero who has powers like Violet from the Disney movie The Incredibles (or if you've never seen that movie), your super power includes creating five unique spherical force field around yourself. Additionally, you can create these force fields around others, no matter where they are just by thinking about it. Each of your force fields have a colorful hue that identifies it and distinguishes each power or blessing you are giving to yourself, your loved ones and everyone you know.

Chapter 5

The Blessing of Safety

Safety—Blue

In your meditation, you are the superhero to all the people you love and care about—everyone you know, and even those you don't know...visualize yourself surrounded by a beautiful, transparent, crystal blue force field that is impenetrable by anything harmful. Bullets bounce off of your force field. Falling objects simply break apart as they crash down around it. Two cars smash into it from either side at once, but there you are, safe and sound in the middle of the smoking wreckage with your blessings because you had your SuperHuman Safety field on. Over-exaggerating the power of the blessing can only make you stronger because it gives you a visual and emotional connection to what you're trying to create. The more energy you have behind it, the stronger your creation.

I think about being safe first when I meditate. Why? I'm sure it has a lot to do with being a parent. I think about my kids standing at my side, healthy and protected from danger. I think about all of us being safe, just safe from harm. I don't imagine horrible situations or anything bad or negative. I just focus on us all being safe. The beauty in doing so is that the magnetic laws that attract all things into your life are based on what you think. I love how best selling author and inspirational leader, Dr. Wayne Dyer says "once you realize that what you think about is what expands...you start getting real careful about what you think about." So I simply meditate on us all being safe. The SuperHuman force field is what keeps us safe.

However, I'm not in denial that bad things happen to people and that sometimes those things cannot be prevented. And I'm not saying that people should be careless or try to stop cars with their bare hands or get in the way of falling trees and so on. Nor am I telling you that there will never be another injury that happens to someone protected by your force field. Rather, I am simply urging you to increase the amount of good and safety you manifest in your life by focusing on fields of safety rather than worrying about what might happen in the future. The fear of the future can be cause people to think very negative thoughts about the unknown, and that is not SuperHuman!

Live SuperHuman Tool: **A SuperHuman power that will help us all is the power to be present, to live and focus on what is happening now without fearfully worrying about the future or living with constant guilt over the past. When you feel guilt, you are living in the past. When you feel fear, you are living in the future. Your super powers come from being present! All your strength is generated by focusing on what you are doing right here, right now.**

Of course you can't ignore your future, nor should you ignore your past. However, by dwelling on it, you will be stuck in a place that is not actual reality. Focus on the future long enough to organize yourself for it and then move on, keeping your mind on what is happening right now. A good example is the gas in your car. You know that you will have to get gas in the future and at that point you will fill up. Until then getting gas in not your primary focus.

In fear you are weak. For example, when do you feel you don't have enough money? Only when you think about the bills and obligations you have or when you feel guilty about the ones you still owe. But right now, this very second as you read these words, what is going on that requires you to need more money? Nothing. If you really think about it, you are simply sitting here reading, not more, not less. No more money than you already have is required. Yes, you may have things you want and bills to pay, but to just sit here and enjoy these words you don't need more than you have. The same goes for safety.

Your present focus on your safety will bring more of it to you and you have no reason to fear the unknown of what is to come. I'd even say that you have more to look forward to by staying present in the now!

One of the best stories I've ever heard about being present is about one of the greatest SuperHumans alive today, Michael Jordan. The story goes: a reporter was trying to get Michael to admit that he is afraid he will miss a game winning shot. Everyone knows that he will take the last shot when the game is on the line, he knows it, his team knows it, the other team knows it, the fans all know it. "That seems like a lot of pressure, aren't you afraid you will miss," the reporter asked. Michael would not give in, and simply said, "Why would I be afraid to miss a shot I haven't taken yet?" This is the powerful presence of a true SuperHuman and a lesson we can all use in our everyday lives.

I'll share with you an example from my own life. My wife and I have some very close friends who often take us out to a very nice dinner. Once we were enjoying a meal together in beautiful Sun Valley, Idaho, and this particular meal was very good, but not nearly as great as some of the meals we had shared with these friends before. After the meal, one of them leaned back and said, "That was literally the best salmon I've ever had." Honestly, I didn't even believe him when he said it but I knew he was being sincere. What I learned from his statement is that he was living in the moment. Even if it wasn't the best salmon ever, it really was the very best salmon in that moment. Now, all my food tastes better because I focus on what I'm eating now, in the moment. Do this and your experience of foods will change forever.

My last and favorite examples of being present are very personal, and I believe that to Live SuperHuman you must find examples like these in your own life that connect you to your present moment. In short, when you need to feel present, these are the things that you will turn to. These are things that you love so much you would do them if you could only choose one or two things to do before you die. These are big ones! One of my favorite things to do in the world is to take my kids to get ice cream cones. I love to watch both my kids eat an ice cream cone so much that I don't even need to get one myself. I have never seen anyone focus on the present moment more intently than those kids right as they are about to take their next bite. It is a spectacular, almost spiritual, thing to witness if you pay close enough attention. I say spiritual because of the deep happiness or bliss, love, surrender, and peace that they feel right in the moment in which they savor every second and taste exactly what they want. The look in their eyes is joyful and content. Their smiles radiate so brightly with such high vibrational frequency that everyone around can't help but be happier simply by being in the presence and power of the whole experience.

When we're getting ice cream, we never talk about concerns they have or about something that happened or something they don't want to happen. We never worry about anything that isn't going to have an effect on us at that moment. The only concern one of the kids may have is about a drip of melted ice cream running down the other side of the cone. Even catching that drip before it makes a mess commands attention on the present moment. If you want a lesson in being present I suggest you take a child to get an ice cream cone. You will learn a valuable life lesson.

Another personal example of feeling focused on the present moment is while making love. It's one of the best ways to become present and to feel what is happening in the now. Let your feeling be your guide. It is hard not to focus on the present moment while making love. If you really enjoy the moment you will savor every feeling you experience. Being present in the moment will allow you greater enjoyment of sex. Additionally, sex gives you some powerful health benefits you may not have been aware of. It relieves stress, boosts your immune system, burns calories, improves cardio-vascular health, creates intimacy, reduces pain, gives you self-esteem, reduces prostate cancer risks, strengthens pelvic floor muscles and helps you sleep better (2). Therefore, the doctor's orders are to eat an ice cream cone and then have sex more frequently to burn off the calories. Hard to argue with a great prescription like that!

Chapter 6

The Blessing of Love

Love—Red

The truth is that I don't really know what else I can say about love that hasn't already been said. Personally, I think the team of writers who wrote the movie Love Actually said it best when they had actor Hugh Grant say the words "love actually is...all around." The truth can't be any plainer than that. It has been said and recognized by the most spiritual people for thousands of years that "love is the greatest power known to man," and "love conquers all." I simply have to agree because there is just no way to really describe it. Love alone defines itself. It functions as a noun, but we all know it as more than that. It is a descriptive term, a feeling, an expression, a sentiment, a powerful force that causes people to do strange things, and so on. Love can define a person's life. One can even create their entire mission, purpose and occupation around love and helping others to understand its power.

I would like to talk about love in terms of how it can be used in your daily life in the same way that I think about love in my meditation. You can take it as far as you want from there. After I have visualized the blue sphere of Safety, I visualize love as a second transparent spherical force field with a red hue that blends with the force field of Safety. It envelops me and protects me, filling me with love, surrounding me with a field of love. I see myself receiving love from all around but I don't need it from any particular source or person. It just is simply all around me at all times. I feel love from the air, the sunshine, the shoes on my feet, the trees rustling in the wind. Even the silence loves me. Of course I feel my beautiful wife sending me love and my super kids pouring out love to me at all times. Everything God has created all came from love and so that is the way I see it.

I simply wish the blessing of love on all the people I can think of, surrounding them like it is surrounding me at all times. I wish they never lack the love they want and always feel loved in abundance. Like anything else, the more love you feel the easier it is to attract! Why not feel yourself surrounded by love all the time and let the perfect love you have hoped for your whole life come easily into your life?! That is much easier than saying how hard it is to find love, or how you wish someone would love you. Once you realize and know that love is yours and comes from you at all times, then attracting love isn't a job or burden anymore. It isn't even a thought, it already exists in your life for you to enjoy. Once you feel love, others will feel how much love you have to give and love that about you. You simply won't be able to stop love from coming at you from all directions.

The reason I feel this is such an important practice for people who want to Live SuperHuman is because it creates self-esteem! The lack of self-esteem has become an epidemic problem in society for many reasons. What matters is the individual solution you can apply in your life right now to help overcome this problem in your life and in the lives of those you love.

Dr. Nathaniel Brandon, one of the greatest SuperHumans alive right now, is the world's leading expert on self-esteem and any one of his books is a must have tool for those who wish to become Super! I have had the privilege of meeting, taking a specialized course from (through Creating Wellness), and even sharing a meal with Dr. Brandon, who is a very sincere, caring individual with a great sense of humor. One of the most important things that he tells people is that "they matter."

There are many definitions for self-esteem and Dr. Brandon's is the best. I simply define it as self-love and the lack of it means not loving yourself enough. Self-love is a behavior that is very learnable and it's something that you'll want to learn as you start to Live SuperHuman.

The sad thing is that many people never learned it as a child and had little practice growing up. Helen, my beautiful, intelligent, sexy wife, who has everything going for her, had to learn it on her own late in life and has come a long way. I'm even still learning because I crave more and more ways to improve. This is a process that requires continuous effort to master and is a life-long endeavor.

Personally, we have raised our kids around the following positive principles so that they create their own self-esteem rather than looking to others to provide it for them. When they do something great like color a picture, make a piece of artwork, or have success in a sport, we don't say "good job." After hearing that external praise "good job," or "great job," or "I'm so proud of you!" thousands of times, what do you think a child, growing into a young adult, looks for to measure themselves? That's right, outside praise and opinions. In the real world those outside opinions can get very critical and harsh very quickly, causing someone to slowly devalue themselves when looking to others for their own self-worth. There is a large body of social research that confirms this. What a horrible thing!

Instead of using externally centered praise, meaning parent-centered (or outside the child), like the examples above, use child-centered praise as demonstrated below.

The parent:

1. Says what they see. "Wow, look at all the colors you used, blue, red, green, yellow, and purple."
2. Notices the effort that got them there. "You must have worked very hard on this." Or "you have been practicing a lot."
3. Ask or state how they feel about themselves in a declarative way. "You must be very proud of yourself." If they say "yes, I am!" respond with something like "I would be, too."

What happens in these three steps is life changing for a person! Suddenly they don't need someone else to tell them that they are loved, great, nice, wonderful, etc. They feel that they are adequate and capable and therefore develop their own self-love, free from the opinions of other people. This can only be taught by someone who truly loves them. Imagine when life gets more complicated and kids get more socially advanced, confused and challenged. If they are less dependent on outside influence to show them love, they will be much, much less likely to turn to outside things like drugs to make themselves feel good. When seeking love they will be much less likely to be hurt by people who are focused on their own needs.

Live SuperHuman Tool: **A child becomes SuperHuman if the parent does three things instead of giving externally focused praise: says what they see, notices effort rather than offering external praise, and asks children how they feel about their accomplishments in a declaratory manner.**

When I think about love, I think of it as a way to fuel my inner fire, so that my super powers can have a greater impact on others. I can magnetize others to me who will help build those powers and also people who can build their own powers through me.

What is beautiful about love is that love is accessible to anyone. It is an eternal power found everywhere in endless abundance. It can be given to others through actions, which fill both the giver and the receiver with love. This is what gives love the magnificence of being a true Super Power.

Below are some of the most famous, beautiful and fun things ever said about love for you to savor. Enjoy!

The Doobie Brothers:
Without love…where would you be now?

The Beatles:
All you need is love.

Nut Brown Hare to Little Nut Brown Hare:
I love you to the moon and back.

I Corinthians 13:4-8
Love always protects, always trusts, always hopes, always perseveres. Love never fails.

Emily Dickinson:
That Love is all there is, is all we know of Love.

The Dalai Lama:
We can live without religion and meditation, but we cannot survive without human affection.

Henry David Thoreau:
There is no remedy for love but to love more.

Martin Luther King, Jr.:
Love is the only force capable of transforming an enemy into friend.

Mary Parrish:
Love vanquishes time.

Mother Teresa:
The hunger for love is much more difficult to remove than the hunger for bread.

And my personal favorite because I've said it to my kids over and over thousands of times since they were babies, simply to make sure they always know that: *I love you 100 percent no matter what.*

Chapter 7

The Blessing of Health

Health—Green

In your meditation, after you visualize the force field of Safety and Love, visualize a vibrant, spherical green force field surrounding you. This green field represents Health. It is what protects you from disease, injury, infirmity, and pain. It heals your body from existing weaknesses and conditions. It helps you focus your mind on what is good and beautiful about your body and how to enhance those qualities. As you focus on those good qualities, the negative qualities or dis-ease will tend to have less magnitude and impact on your health. When I visualize the SuperHuman field of Health, I visualize a green grid, like a screen of lasers that is so tight not even a virus could fit through the screen. This screen passes through my body from head to toe zapping anything bad and healing problems like nerve subluxations, cancer, oxidized cholesterol build up in my blood vessels, viruses, bad bacteria, sprained ligaments, injuries, toxins and so on. I visualize the screen eliminating and pushing out anything in my body that contributes to ill health. I also visualize this screen passing through everyone else I can think of at the same time. It is my way of sending good energy focused on health to others, and I love to do it.

One thing I want for people, more than anything else, is for them to have fantastic, supercharged health. My heart aches knowing how much needless suffering goes on with people. Health is not complicated, I promise! I will prove it to you in this Section 3 of the book, which is my favorite section already.

As a doctor, educator, and student of wellness, you have to know that I am very excited to share the secrets that I have known for many years and shared with thousands of people in my daily practice! I realize the irony of calling these daily lifestyle practices "secrets" in today's world, which is filled with so much good information. However, there is bad information, like quick fix claims, medical dogma, and played out health schemes, ideas and products. Good or bad, these things all contribute to the greater consciousness of health on the planet and the attention each individual places on wellness. The good news—no, the great news—is that much of what has come to the surface of healthcare in the past few years has been the realization that our current system is in serious need for an overhaul! What you are going to find out here is that in order to overhaul the system, the philosophical beliefs that created the system will have to change.

In recent years, modern medicine has been identified by intelligent researchers at prestigious institutions such as Johns Hopkins University, as the number one killer of Americans above cancer and heart disease. This research study was published in Life Extension Magazine and received quite a lot of press only a few years ago. The top medical killers identified were as follows:

Condition	Deaths	Cost	Author
Adverse Drug Reactions	106,000	$12 billion	Lazarou, Suh
Medical error	98,000	$2 billion	IOM
Bedsores	115,000	$55 billion	Xakellis, Barczak
Infection	88,000	$5 billion	Weinstein, MMWR
Malnutrition	108,800	———	Nurses Coalition
Outpatients	199,000	$77 billion	Starfield, Weingart
Unnecessary Procedures	37,136	$122 billion	HCUP
Surgery-Related	32,000	$9 billion	AHRQ
TOTAL	**783,936**	**$282 billion**	

Life Extension 2006 (3)

Once secretive, many drug company insiders have broken free from the stranglehold of their company and spoken out against dangerous practices, sales and marketing techniques to consumers, as well as foul politics. Did you know that there are more drug company lobbyists in Washington, D.C., than there are congressmen? These companies have tried to pass laws that would force people to take medication, vaccinations, or cancer treatment against their will. Can you imagine being told by a legal official that you will go to jail and have your child taken from you if you choose not to have them drugged a certain way? This craziness has already happened to some, and this type of nightmare is only possible when you have enormous financial power to force these types of beliefs, judgments and regulations into society.

In 2008, for the first time in history, lifestyle disease surpassed infectious illness as the leading cause of death world-wide. This is an extraordinary thing to comprehend! Think about it, deaths attributed to obesity, cardiovascular disease, and some say even cancer, which can all be preventable with healthy lifestyle, now outnumber death by malaria, yellow fever, AIDS, and so on. This is a catastrophic blow to the health of the world, and at the same time an enormous clarion call for leadership and individual action for health and wellness of the people and planet.

I believe that The 5 Blessings are critical to moving the health and wellness of the world in the right direction. One of the core ways people can start using these blessings is through the blessing of happiness.

Chapter 8

The Blessing of Happiness

Happiness—Yellow

I would like to start this section by declaring that I believe happiness is one of the strongest superpowers any SuperHuman can have. After you have visualized the green field of health and given it as a blessing to everyone you know, visualize a yellow force field forming around you, blending into the blue, red and green of your existing blessings of safety, love and health. The brightness of the yellow field is representative of the bright, vibrant energy of happiness.

Did you know that all of your moods have a different energy level that can be measured scientifically? This is some of the astonishing research that's ever been done. It's called the measurement of subtle energies. Subtle energies are energies that don't follow the typical laws of physics as we understand them. These energies are so small, so hard to measure, that only as scientific technology gets more and more advanced are we able to even detect them and start to study how these energies affect our lives. We all know they exist, consciously or subconsciously because we sense them all the time. These feelings are things like our moods or our energy levels or our Chi, or life force, as the Chinese call it.

Some amazing research has been done on people's moods and how it affects the moods of other people. Would you believe me if

I told you that your happiness has a direct effect on the happiness of your siblings, your neighbors, and the people around you? Well believe it because this research shows the first clues into how our energy levels and our happiness affect those of the people around us. A research paper published in the British Medical Journal in 2008 titled "Happiness May Be Contagious" states that people's happiness can be influenced by those who they are connected to whether they know them or not. The researchers found that your emotional state may depend upon the emotional experience of those you don't even know who are 2 or 3 degrees removed from you. People can "catch" emotional states that are found in other individuals and "the effect isn't just fleeting," study investigator Nicholas Christakis, MD, PhD, from Harvard Medical School stated. When an individual becomes happy, a friend living within a mile receives a 25 percent increase in their own happiness. A co resident spouse receives an 8 percent increase. Siblings living within a mile of each other receive a 14 percent increase and neighbors a 34 percent increase (3). This is amazing! If you still aren't convinced, this study included 4739 individuals and more than 50,000 social and family ties!!! And if you ask me, it proves my theory that sending blessings to people that are filled with positive energy can do nothing but good for those around us and even across the globe as demonstrated by the study we talked about earlier on by Dr. Emoto.

I believe that anyone who is a happy person, has a positive outlook, and really looks forward to what is coming next in life, is an expert on happiness. We can all learn something from people who have these qualities. The truth is that everyone has a past with some combination of problems. From family issues that have caused you life long stress, to some type of abuse leading to self-esteem issues, or simple mistakes that you are not proud of, we all have something that we are not proud of. What I want you to think about is this: Why does my life stink so bad? As one of my favorite teachers, Dr. Wayne Dyer puts it, "we all have this big sack of manure we call our past that we carry around with us. And every once in a while we stop, we set it down, open it up, and reach way down in there and pull some out. Then we smear it all over ourselves and wonder, 'why does my life stink so bad?"

To me this is a powerful truth and it goes right to the point we discussed earlier about being in the present moment. Whenever you live in the now, right now, it is much easier to be super happy. When you go to the past or the future you make things much more difficult because they are unknowns to the now. It's easy to be happy about the now because it is what you know you can focus on and be a part of for sure. Think about when you get a present. You are happy partly because you are focused on that moment only. The unexpected gift of something you want or need makes everyone happy! If you are happy, then give yourself the present every moment you possibly can. It will always be easier to be happy when you do this.

Know Your Business

"Dr. Rook, I really want to be happy but there are lots of things about my personal relationships that really make it hard for me to be happy all the time." Unfortunately, this is an all too common statement. It could mean a relationship with a parent, sibling, friend or even a child, creates continual stressful wear and tear on you. Does this resemble something that has gone on in your life? If so, let's analyze this statement together. First of all, when you say "I really want to be happy but..." you are giving up all of your personal control and power. What you are saying here is that your happiness is not up to you but it's up to somebody else. Don't ever do this! You are severely damaging your self-esteem. It's very difficult, or impossible, for anyone to be happy when all of their power is surrendered to other people. As SuperHumans, giving up your power is against your code.

Now I know I can't just say, "Hey, snap out of it!" If it were that simple you would've already done it. This is a very important place to start, however, because before you can start giving these gifts to other people in a genuine way, and be authentic to yourself, you will want to develop the superpower blessing of happiness for yourself.

Breaking this down further... "personal relationships that really make it hard" is the next section we want to analyze. When we say personal relationships we're talking about people who are very close to us, usually a mother or father, sibling, girlfriend or boyfriend, husband or wife. In some part of us deep down we all want to have the strongest happiest closest personal relationships in these areas. However, for some reason in life many of our challenges are brought to us by the people who are closest to us. I have heard it said that we choose a mate based on how much this person will challenge us or make us grow. If we choose our mates based on something we learned from our parents then we could even say that we are trying to solve issues created by our parents that we haven't figured out yet. I don't know if all this is true but I will say that just recognizing these possibilities is a step in the right direction.

Being honest with yourself is so important because it gives you the freedom to move. When you constantly deceive to yourself about who you are or where you're at in your life, it's impossible to make any meaningful change and move forward.

I'm going to share a very powerful tool with you that will help you address personal problems or challenges you have already faced as well as those that you may face in the future. It will help you address your unhappiness so that you can focus on promoting your happiness.

Live SuperHuman Tool: **Always be honest with yourself and with others.**

Being honest with yourself means you acknowledge the fact that you have something to do with your own unhappiness. It also means that you don't place blame on anybody else for your own unhappiness. Your relationships don't all have to be perfect. It isn't necessary for you to have harmonious, loving relationships with everyone on the planet. As a matter of fact, no matter how loving and wonderful you may be, there will be people who just don't jibe with you or even like you. That may even be a family member. Guess what? **That isn't your business, concern or problem.** That is their business. Their feelings about you are what they think and how they feel and it is only under their control. You can't think for another person, you can't decide for another person, and you can't act for another person. You can only control what you think, feel, say and do. And this is your business.

This is one of the greatest lessons I've ever learned, and I want you to commit to learning it right now! What other people think about you is their business. You can't control it in any way. You cannot do anything to change what others think and it isn't even your job to change it. Your job is to be true to your purpose, your SuperHuman code, and **mind your own business!** This means you don't need to focus any energy on what someone else thinks about you. It is a waste of your energy to do so. Of course this does not mean you shouldn't heed good feedback, advice or constructive criticism from bosses, coworkers, or coaches. What it means is gain an understanding and filter for what to internalize and utilize from others and what not to. As a doctor taking care of thousands of people, of course there are times when I am not the right doctor for someone because it just isn't a good fit. The first time I found out that somebody didn't like me as their doctor it hurt my feelings and I was upset. Who isn't upset when you find out somebody doesn't like you the way you want to be liked? Over time what I realized is that just because I'm not the right doctor for someone doesn't mean I can't love them or that I'm a bad person. It just means I'm not the right doctor and that's not personal for me. It is a personal decision for them and that's good. That means they are being honest with themselves. Of course, I do everything I can to let that person know I will help them find a doctor that works for them, but whatever they say or think about me when they leave is not my business, and therefore not for me to feel good or bad about.

The very best book I have ever read on being honest with yourself is called "Loving What Is" by Byron Katie. In her book Ms. Katie teaches readers all about knowing your own business and knowing other people's business. She discusses whose business to pay attention to and whose business to ignore. She also teaches the simplest and most incredible tool to help someone process and handle psychological stress. That tool is called The Work, and it's the most effective tool I've ever used personally—other than a chiropractic adjustment. The Work is a short, simple process of challenging your thoughts about any issue, typically ones that cause you negative stress, so that you can understand and eliminate what really is causing you the painful stress.

It is very important for you as a developing SuperHuman to acquire as many tools as possible to help you handle, build your defenses against, and process out psychological stress that accumulates in your life because stress leads to unhappiness.

One thing you must understand about psychological stress and stress in general, is that stress has a cumulative effect. It does not come in and then go away. It tends to build up on your body. Your central nervous system is the part of your body responsible for perceiving stresses and then adapting your body to the stresses so that you can effectively handle them. For example, if your nervous system perceives information that you are cold or have a chill, then your nervous system will send signals to your muscles, your skin and your hair follicles to give you goose bumps and eventually start to shiver to help warm you up. This is a classic example of your nervous system doing its number one job—adaptation. The better at adapting you are, the longer, higher quality of life you will have.

Live SuperHuman Tool: **The two best tools to help free your body from the negative effects of emotional stress are chiropractic care and questioning your thoughts about anything that causes you negative stress.**

Having tools to make sure your central nervous system is working as close to optimal as possible is a critical thing that you must do to Live SuperHuman.

Chapter 9

The Blessing of Prosperity

Prosperity—Purple

Safety, Love, Health and Happiness lead you to the final blessing of your meditation, the purple field of prosperity. Visualize this force field surrounding you, becoming one with the four other brightly lit blessings, adding purple to the mix. You may have noticed that prosperity gets a lot of lip service. It's difficult as a regular "Joe" to listen to people talk about prosperity when you constantly struggle to make ends meet on a day-to-day basis. I know this as well as anyone else.

When I set out to open my practice at 23 years old, I had a couple thousand dollars to my name and more than $100,000 in debt. I was recently married, had a 2 year old daughter and newborn son, and the economy was crashing shortly after the 9/11 World Trade Center attacks. I was also bullheaded and had my own ideas about how I wanted to run my practice and no other doctor seemed to offer what I wanted. I was under a lot of pressure, but I had been told by mentors and gurus that I had all the tools: a good education at the right school, an up-beat personality, and the gift of good communication. I was told that if I told the truth, stayed enthusiastic and did a good job, I would be successful, and prosperity would come to me. I was told that it was 100 percent up to me.

Up to that point in my life, nothing had been very difficult. I had always gotten good grades in school without struggling. I was an excellent athlete and excelled at any sport. I had a lawn mowing business that bought me two jet skis and a truck and allowed me to spend extra time with my dad. I always had money in the bank and never really wanted for anything. My family all got along very well and I was close with my brother and sister.

I knew what success was and what it felt like. Really, I had never tasted defeat in my life. When I was told that all I would have to do was keep doing my thing and I would be successful, I believed it. That was truth for me. For some people it may happen that way, but I can tell you that it doesn't happen that way for everyone, and it certainly didn't for me. I did exactly as I was coached to do by mentors. I even hired consultants and spent over $100,000 over the next 5 years learning ways become a better doctor and a better business person. My business started to grow and I did start to experience some success. I was able to genuinely help people in ways I had always dreamed of. But I was starting from scratch and no matter how hard I worked to grow my business, it never took off the way I had hoped it would... the way I knew it could.

You must never do one thing I did. I began comparing myself and the speed of my success in business to the way that other doctors' businesses had succeeded. When you compare yourself to others, you break your SuperHuman code. You break rule number one because you give up your power by putting your energy into what others are doing instead of putting energy into what you are doing. You begin paying attention to their business instead of minding your own business. The end result for you will always be catastrophic. I learned the hard way.

Eventually my debts mounted and so did my stresses. The weight of it all became harder and harder on my marriage. After five years, I was divorced and living with my mom in her three bedroom house. All I had after the divorce was my business and its hefty expenses, my debt, my clothes, and two couches. I didn't even have a bed! It was not how I anticipated my life going. After all, I was told I'd be very successful.

I'm not talking about success in terms of visualizing, dreaming and setting goals or manifesting your destiny in an energetic or spiritual context. I'm talking about setting goals you specifically intend to achieve and manifesting them through determination, action and through a SuperHuman will to stay consistent. The only way to build a beautiful home, skyscraper or life is with a blueprint to guide your actions. A specific plan of action that tells you exactly where all the pieces of the puzzle will go to lead you to the finished product. Imagine what building a home would be like with no plans or blueprints…it would be impossible.

After sleeping on a couch every night for months trying to pull yourself up out of a hole, you realize quickly that you are at a turning point. This turning point, right here right now in this moment reading this book, is when and where you realize that you have the power to drive things in the direction you want them to go. I didn't know how long it was going to take to get off my couch, and I didn't know how fast it would happen. I didn't even know what I wanted to achieve, but I knew that I was going in one direction and one direction only. Up and out of the hole. In order to do that, I had my business, my self-confidence and my surprisingly intact happiness, and I knew that I could do what I had set out to achieve originally by redefining what success means to me.

What I came to realize is that the tools I thought would bring me success in business were the tools that actually benefitted me the most in a personal way in a difficult time in my life. Those tools may not have grown my business the way I had hoped they would, but that really wasn't as important as keeping myself a happy person who cares for others. That the essence of being SuperHuman is taking lessons like that and making something out of them. And that became my new definition of success: When you are challenged, allow the true colors of your character to shine and take you in a new direction.

At the same time I realized my definition of success was evolving, things began to change. I fell in love with my amazing wife, Helen, and really started to focus on the direction I wanted to go. These changes in my life led to what I consider my prosperity.

The terms *success* and *prosperity* are not necessarily interchangeable, however, no matter which term you are talking about, I believe that money, or finances play a role in both. The best way you can help yourself and the world is by being able to contribute. The more resources you have to draw from, the more you are able to give and help others. If you constantly need help and have limited resources and finances, it is very difficult to give and contribute on a consistent basis.

We are all aware that with more money, you have the ability to do things that lack of money does not provide. You can donate, volunteer, start a business, create jobs, and not to mention have less stress. Financial struggle is one of the biggest causes of negative Neuro-Spiritual stress. I've read that over 50 percent of divorce is caused by financial lack straining a marriage. I believe it. I've been there. Another of the most painful things I noticed during times of financial struggle was the horrible feeling of inability to give to others. I always gave my time and services abundantly even if it was not easy on my finances. In reality, it is okay to be selfish when you need to be. To protect yourself and your family is critical. Don't be hard on yourself. Be honest with yourself and ask who and how can you help the most right now, no matter where you are financially.

"Wisdom is the seed of gratitude. It blossoms as generosity and that's just a start. The fruit of generosity is prosperity. And true prosperity is a grateful heart."

- Pat Mc Donald

My hope is that through this book, you make your way to a higher level of financial prosperity so you can make your family more comfortable, create and give to others so that we all can rise up together. Upcoming in The 3 Elements of Wellness and chapters that follow, you will find ways in which you can begin to form your personal blueprint or even solidify it by filling in potential gaps. Remember the weakest link phenomenon as you read on: just as a chain will always fail at its weakest link, no matter where you are in life, your life will be held back, or breakdown, where your personal weakest link exists.

Live SuperHuman Tool: The 5 Blessings are a legitimate, simple and powerful way you can consistently enhance your well being. Use these tools as described to raise your own wellness and those around you.

With all the current consumer awareness, education, and desire, new diets are popping up constantly. Health products are becoming more and more profuse and confusing. The paradox is that even though the message of wellness is more abundant than ever, which is a very good thing, people are still puzzled when it comes to what specific, customized actions to take to help themselves adjust their blueprint to be more well. In other words, people know they are slightly unique physically and functionally and they need to do something, but they don't know what things will be right for their body.

But which diet is best to build my blueprint? That is the question! I want you to know that there is a little known secret about which one of these diets is best. It's well known among elite professionals within the health and wellness industry, and I'll reveal that secret to you in chapters 14 and 15.

There are countless supplements on the market and tons of questions as to which ones are the best. I will clear the air on which supplements you should be taking in chapter 16.

How about exercise programs, yoga, stretching and choosing doctors? Which ways should you really be taking care of yourself? Great questions! I will address all these issues for you in the upcoming pages. I'll also tell you one more thing right now: all this information is already out there, and my goal is to bring it together for you. I'm simply going to put all the information together for you so, that you know what to do, you know how to do it and you know who you can trust for accurate information. Think of me as your most trusted SuperHuman Wellness Professional, who is about to give you a blueprint of the new healthcare developed especially for SuperHumans and those who want to become SuperHuman!

Remember your blessings to have and to give:
Safety-Blue. Be blessed with protection from harm.
Love-Red. Be blessed with the greatest power ever known.
Health-Green. Be blessed with a strong body and mind.
Happiness-Yellow. Be blessed with laughter and bliss.
Prosperity-Purple. Be blessed with the lifestyle of your dreams.

Section 3

Physical
Bio-chemical
Neuro-spiritual

Chapter 10

The 3 SuperHuman Elements of Wellness

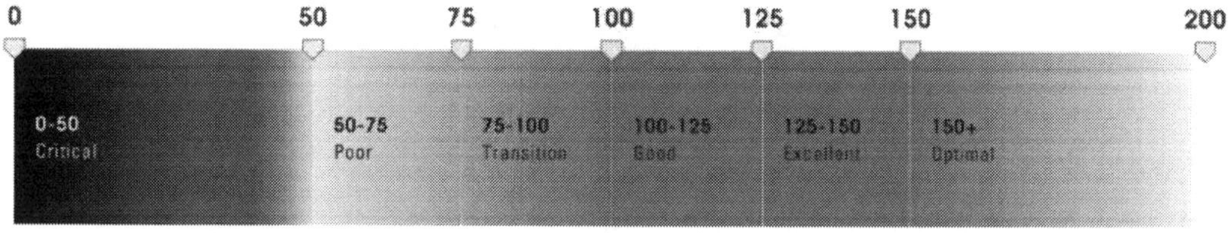

Live SuperHuman Tool: **Use this scale to identify your level of wellness right now. Pick a spot on the scale where you think you are and circle it. Zero represents ill health or death and 200 is the most optimal level of wellness you can imagine for yourself. What matters is not where actually are, but where you think you are on the scale. And no matter where you actually are, you can always do better. The SuperHuman Elements of Wellness will help move you to higher levels of well being. Read on!**

With so many types of diets and so much seemingly conflicting advice out there, it can be hard to know what the right choice is. What do you eat, how do you exercise, should you stretch, what about supplements? I'm here to help you answer those questions and more. Think of me as your personal, and most trusted, SuperHuman Wellness Professional. I will address all of these issues in the upcoming chapters. But first, to make things even easier, we will break the health section down in to three, easy to follow, parts. Your health is made up of three interconnected elements: Physical, Bio-chemical, and Neuro-spiritual.

Physical means what you do with your body, or how physically fit you are.
Bio-Chemical means what you put in your body and how you eat.
Neuro-Spiritual means how you think and believe and how you act due to those beliefs.

To become truly SuperHuman you must improve your wellness in all three elements at once. Think of each element as having a score from zero to one hundred. Each score must go up at the same time, all elements lifting one another, to get to true wellness. If you put a lot of focus on "diet and exercise," you may have a Physical fitness score of 90 and a Bio-Chemical score of 85, but your Neuro-spiritual score may be a lousy 50, which is why you always struggle to stay consistently healthy and fit. If that's the case, you will constantly go back and forth between exercising and eating well, and failing to keep it up. What weighs on you mentally is what will constantly drag you down. The weakest link is always the one that breaks the chain and prevents you from reaching your goals. We'll talk about how to prevent that chain from breaking.

Chapter 11

Physical Element: Strength

Strength

Physical health refers to the way you keep your body fit. How your body physically looks and how you move your body to keep it physically fit. Simply put, this is how you exercise. Many different kinds of workouts improve your fitness and it can be quite a confusing journey to find a solution that works for you. If you've ever tried to find a work out program on DVD or in a book, then you know what I'm talking about. When you go to the book store, there are hundreds of books on fitness and how to work out! Hundreds! Some talk about weight lifting, some running, some do exercises with balls, some with bands, some with difficult or expensive equipment and so on.

Most workout facilities like gyms are a great place to get fit and you can have lots of fun doing it, but you have to follow through a few times per week. I have two memberships at different facilities, which allows me to have even more convenient access to be able to work out at the gym of my choice. More convenience means more use any way you slice it. You don't have to be crazy like me and have multiple memberships, however, location and ease of access is the most important factor when choosing your gym membership.

A gym is not the only place to get fit. There are many ways to start, like simply walking or biking. Unfortunately all those options are also what give some people the perception that fitness is complicated. I can tell you, from the perspective of a doctor who works with the physical aspect of the human body every day, that physical health is not difficult at all. I will simplify what you need right now.

You only need to strengthen three things for SuperHuman physical health:

1. Strengthen muscles for moving your body.
2. Strengthen your heart muscle.
3. Strengthen your flexibility, movement and alignment.

That's it! There is no big secret here and there are only so many ways to accomplish those goals.

Here is a super secret that I'll bet you never thought of before. Did you know that muscles only do one job? That's right, the only job they have is to contract. That's it. They don't have a mind of their own, they don't have a "memory," or go into spasm, or become all knotted up all by themselves with no outside influence. If muscles only contract, and they have no ability to do so on their own with no outside influence, then what tells a muscle to contract? That's right, the brain and nerve system. Each muscle has nerves that connect to it, sending signals when to contract. When that signal turns off, the muscle then rests and can elongate again. The nerves that connect to your muscles are connected to other nerves that eventually make it back to the spinal cord and the up to the brain. Every muscle movement that you have is the result of a nerve signal, most of which originated in the brain.

This process is vitally important to realize in your daily life because it affects you in many ways. Have you ever noticed that if you have knot in a muscle and you try to rub it out, or get a massage, it may feel great for a short time but it eventually comes back? Of course you have, we all have knots like this at times. But the muscle is not the source of the problem, it is simply doing what it is told to do by your nerve system. Your spinal posture may have bad movement and poor alignment causing nerve stress, or subluxations, and those aching muscles are the result of bracing, or protecting your spine so that more nerve damage is not created. Rubbing that muscle will feel great because the muscle is working very hard and it would love a rest, however, unless the misalignment and subluxation is fixed, that muscle will continue to be tight doing its job. Not until you see a doctor whose expertise is in removing that nerve stress can your muscles begin to relax fully. Working on the muscles with massage and exercise will simply speed up the muscle relaxing and healing process for you after the subluxation is corrected. That is why chiropractic care is your first Live SuperHuman tool for this chapter.

Live SuperHuman Tool: **Chiropractors are the only doctors who correct subluxations, or nerve disturbance, restoring proper communication in the central nervous system. Healthy nerve communication will then produce healthier function in your organs, cells and systems.**

Another area in which improved nerve communication can have a positive impact is in your strengthening exercise. Most people think strength is gained by muscles growing and becoming larger. This is true, but it mostly happens in men and it only happens after the muscle becomes more fully activated. Most daily activities like lifting a sandwich or glass of water only requires a small portion of muscle fibers in your biceps muscle to be activated. This is not a difficult, tiring or strenuous task for a healthy muscle. However, when you do a job like lifting heavy weights over and over, focusing just on your biceps muscles, it requires the nerve system to activate more fibers in the muscle to gain the strength needed. This is really important because your nerve system needs to be healthy to perform this job. Therefore, most initial strength gain from working out comes from nerves activating more of your muscles, not muscles growing larger. This is also the primary way that women gain strength.

Building muscle strength requires your body to constantly burn calories. This will help you boost your metabolism which will cause you to lose weight more easily, if this is your goal. All of this muscle strength gain will have a huge impact on your health and vitality, especially if the strength gained is in your heart muscle.

Strengthening your heart muscle is critical to becoming SuperHuman. Exercise that improves cardiovascular fitness will lengthen your life and decrease your risk for many diseases. This is the best way to burn calories quickly and get your body strong and vital.

Cardio exercise is very important for digestive motility and intestine function, helping your digestive system stay healthy. Cardio can also help you sleep more soundly and wake up feeling energized instead of drained. A variety of cardiovascular exercise will work wonders to strengthen your heart. A brisk walk for 20 minutes, 3-4 times every week is the easiest way to get started. More advanced cardio exercises are swimming, jogging, aerobic classes ranging from dance to kickboxing, and so on. Many gyms offer these kinds of classes, and I always recommend getting some type of professional help if you are not sure what is good for you specifically. Chiropractors are perfect doctors to offer this type of wellness advising in addition to a personal trainer or local fitness expert.

Live SuperHuman Tool: **Build muscle strength 3 different ways to help lose weight!**

One last thing you can do to burn off calories is so simple you might have never thought of it: fidget. People who are "fidgeters" can burn nearly double the calories each day compared to people who hold still. Even if both of them go to the gym for an equally long cardio work out. For example, people who stand or pace while they talk on the phone instead of sit burn many more calories. Instead of just standing in line simply shift your weight back and forth, left to right. You could squeeze one of those squishy stress balls while you are sitting and thinking, or in a meeting.

I can see it now you are in a meeting nervously watching your boss pacing back and forth as you anticipate his next words. Meanwhile, you are squeezing a ball or shifting your feet to fidget and burn calories. As the tension builds you see your boss take notice of the copy of this book you happen to have on the table next to you. Suddenly your boss looks over at you and asks, "becoming SuperHuman?" You nod, and he or she says, "good, me too!" then continues the meeting. How fun, and yet you are both on common ground to make your team stronger. Maybe you'll even get a raise!

Chapter 12

Flexibility, Movement and Alignment

Strengthen your Flexibility, Movement and Alignment

While strengthening your muscles, it is important to keep them flexible. One of the most overlooked areas in fitness can be flexibility. The Mayo Clinic recognizes these major benefits from stretching and flexibility:

- **Flexibility increases power.** Flexible muscles improve performance. Daily tasks such as lifting, bending or hurrying become easier and less tiring.
- **Flexibility improves joint range of motion.** Good range of motion keeps you in better balance. This will help keep you on your feet and less prone to injury from falls as you age.
- **Flexibility improves circulation.** Improving flexibility increases blood flow to your muscles. Improved circulation can reduce recovery time after injuries.
- **Flexibility promotes better posture.** Improving flexibility keeps your muscles in a healthier tone, allowing you to maintain proper posture and minimize aches and pains.
- **Flexibility can relieve stress.** Good flexibility relaxes the tense muscles that often accompany stress.
- **Flexibility may help prevent injury.** Preparing your muscles and joints for activity can protect you from injury, especially if your muscles or joints are tight

Live SuperHuman Tool: **Strengthen flexibility to ease suffering with pain and tell everyone know how you felt better through increased flexibility. Use the resources in this chapter to implement LS code principles 2 (always share your powers with as many people as possible) and 3 (always help others, and the world, whenever you can)!**

I have come to believe that many so-called "facts" about stretching are myths. The reason I claim that is because we have to define stretching. Stretching that would give you the benefits listed above would have to lengthen your muscles, which is what most people believe they are doing when they stretch. The fact is that it's not that simple. Let me explain.

The school of thought by most of the world's leading experts in exercise physiology, training and rehab protocols of world-class athletes is that stretching the old-fashioned way does not actually lengthen your muscles. If this is true, then stretching could actually be very bad for you in terms of making you more prone to injuries. The new science of athletic performance used by doctors and trainers of elite athletes around the world says that stretching the old-fashioned way stretches your ligaments and tendons making them more prone to injury and damage. Many athletes such as Olympians and pro football and baseball players have struggled with injuries that have plagued their careers for years and many of them have done tons of stretching. You might ask how that could be given all of their top-notch training and exercise programs. That is a very good question that has been asked by some very intelligent experts.

Muscles don't actually stretch very easily. When stretched, a muscle will actually contract to resist the stretching and the potential damage to itself. Muscles have one job that happens two ways. Contraction is the only function of muscles. One type of contraction is a shortening contraction, or concentric contraction. The second type of contraction is a lengthening contraction, or eccentric contraction. Muscles work in pairs. While one shortens, the other in the pair elongates. A shortening contraction occurs when you want to pull or push something or use a muscle to perform an act that requires strength. When that happens, the opposite muscle is given a signal by your nervous system to elongate, or perform an eccentric contraction.

One theory purports that all athletic injury comes from a muscle's inability to absorb force. If a force or shock hits a part of the body, the muscle's job is to contract quickly and to be super strong in order protect the body from injury. Of course if you get hit by a truck there is no way you can train to handle that kind of force. If the muscle cannot react fast enough to absorb the force, then a tendon, ligament or bone will have to absorb that force and that will cause injury. Of course, the question is why didn't the muscle react fast enough?

The answer to that question goes back to the nervous system and subluxations. If you have a subluxation, which is a disturbance or blockage in the nerve signal to or from the brain, then the signal won't arrive in time or with a clear message. This is another time you'll need a chiropractor to fix the subluxation in order to get proper muscle training.

The training and warm-up programs for most Olympic and professional athletes are transitioning from old-fashioned stretching, like touching your toes without bouncing for 15-25 seconds, into a newer high-tech way of lengthening your muscles. Old-fashioned stretching is no longer recommended on the day of the event. Instead, athletes engage in activities that warm-up their muscles and get them ready for an event or explosive activities. For example, I like to play basketball 3 to 4 days every week. In the past, to get ready for a game I would have made sure to stretch my legs thoroughly before playing. Denis Thompson, injury rehab specialist to literally thousands of professional athletes and developer of the ARP Trainer, offers new recommendations for warming up. Thompson advocates that instead of stretching to warm-up we should simply warm-up by doing explosive activities like jogging, jumping, and running that prepare muscles for the game we're about to play. An Olympic volleyball player or gymnast would do the same thing to prepare them for their game or event that day. Stretching exercises should only be done in preparation or on practice days but not on game days. This is the *new school* way injuries are being prevented and performance enhanced.

The spectacular technology called the ARP Trainer (or ARP) can also help someone who has any injury or pain recover more quickly and possibly avoid surgery. ARP stands for Accelerated Recovery Performance and applies a new philosophy to injury treatment. Typical injury treatment is based on this 4 step process: decrease swelling, increase mobility, increase strength, and then decrease compensation—in that order. You have heard the old saying...RICE; rest, ice, compression, elevation.

ARP injury treatment attacks the last step in the process first and pays maximum attention to eliminating compensation. Applying the ARP quickly identifies which muscles are primarily involved in compensating for the injury. Gentle electrical stimulation is applied to those muscles to produce an overload and forces the muscles to go back to normal and stop compensating. Healthy patterns of muscle activity are what allow the muscles to stop compensating.

The combination of learning healthy muscle activity and the unique effects of the ARP allows all 4 steps in the healing process to be treated simultaneously assisting someone to heal at a much faster rate! Compensation to injuries is counterproductive to healing and can get in the way of the healing process. Addressing the compensation right away is what allows the ARP Trainer to get such fast results. When I say fast, I mean unbelievably fast! The clinic shows results for recovery rates at 60-80 percent faster than traditional conservative care. For example, with the ARP Trainer, pulled muscles can heal in just 8-12 days as opposed to the more than 8-week recovery it might take. Sprains can heal in 3-5 days instead of 6-8 weeks. Torn ACLs in the knee can be repaired without surgery. Spinal disk injuries heal without surgery or months of suffering in pain! Unbelievable? Well believe it. The company even has a guarantee!

If you have been suffering from an injury or any kind of pain that you are tired of, I strongly encourage you to go to LiveSuperHuman.com and contact the ARP Clinic. You have nothing to lose and they can typically help you in 10 sessions or less. You don't even have to be there to receive this recovery treatment! The ARP professionals have perfected an incredible system to send the ARP Trainer machine directly to you and help you at home through live web video. The first time I heard all of this information I literally didn't believe it.

Then after meeting Mr. Thompson and finding out that they have the most comprehensive list of professional athletes as clients I've ever seen, including over 500 NFL players, over 200 MLB, NHL and NBA players, and countless professional Olympic athletes. After speaking to the chiropractor for the New England Patriots and listening to him verify all of this information, I was a believer.

Live SuperHuman Tool: **Use the Accelerated Recovery Performance Trainer to help heal injuries and eliminate pain.**

Now you have the benefit of knowing not only how important flexibility is, but the best way to achieve flexibility. All you have to do is put together a program to strengthen your muscles and your heart and increase your flexibility. The big trick is how to get it done easily, comfortably, quickly and while having fun so that you will continue to do it. Many people join a gym and go occasionally but can't make a special trip all the time get there. Of course, some people never go at all. If you work out and are committed but can't seem to make it all the time because you travel or just want to do your workout at home, I have a great solution for you! If you would prefer to work out at home all the time, I have a super solution for you! Or, if you would like a home program to get you on the right path so that you can then feel good about joining a gym, I have super solution for you too!

I have developed an exercise program that incorporates beautiful movements and coordination from martial arts, the resistance training from weights, and the flexibility training from Yoga. Combine that with some cardiovascular heart pumping, and you have a full body workout that not only strengthens your muscles, heart and flexibility, but will burn calories, and boost your metabolism, decreasing the need for extra fat storage, and help you look and feel great...even SuperHuman!

From all this research, and years of experience (and of course with some help), I have developed a totally unique, simple, beautiful, and fun exercise routine that you can do everyday and enjoy. A brand new invention called the SuperStretch Towel is what makes this possible. The SuperStretch Towel (SST) was invented specifically to help improve strength and flexibility. An entirely new category of stretching has even been developed around the SST because it makes flexibility exercises that used to have to be performed with two people possible by yourself! Also the SST's elastic ability allows you to build muscle with resistance exercise like lifting weights. Each SST comes with all the programs you need for strengthening your muscles, heart, and flexibility. Go to LiveSuperHuman.com to learn more and there you can even expand your fitness program with various tips and updates as well.

Live SuperHuman Tool: **Use the SuperStretch Towel program to get and stay super fit.**

Thousands of SuperHumans already use SST's. Professional golfers use it and hundreds of doctors recommend SST's to their patients. The new Live SuperHuman fitness program is designed to be more comfortable, more convenient, take less time and get better results than old-fashioned programs offer. If this sounds like it interests you, then I invite you to take part and take action.

Live SuperHuman Tool: **SuperHumans don't hesitate, they act! Before now, many opportunities to improve your life have been ignored. Just like super heroes act quickly to save someone's life, it is even more important SuperHumans act quickly to save their own lives! If you don't save your own life now, you will be no good to anybody else later.**

Chapter 13

SuperHuman Elements of Wellness: BioChemical

Bio-Chemical

The term bio-chemical refers to what goes into your body. It's everything you put in your body, as well as everything your body absorbs from your environment. This includes foods, supplements, medications, pollutants and toxins of any kind in lotions detergents or make-up. All chemicals that enter your body affect your biology, directly impacting the quality of your life. Thus, the term Bio-Chemical.

Did you know that it is estimated your body performs over 6 trillion chemical reactions every second?! Even more amazing is the fact that each chemical reaction is directly governed by your brain and nerve system in one way or another. That means that every chemical reaction is interdependent upon every other chemical reaction to keep you alive and functioning well. Six trillion chemical reactions each second sounds like a lot but when you consider your body is made up of over 100 trillion cells that means only 6 percent of your cells are actually told to produce a chemical change each second. I say "told to" because cells are kind of like little soldiers who carry out orders. When the central nerve system gives an order, only then can it be carried out by a part of your body like a cell.

What does this mean to you and me? It means two things—two very important things. First, it means **you had better have a healthy central nerve system getting messages clearly and easily to your body**. Second, it means **you had better have very good, protective and healthy nutrients in your body at all times**. If you don't have both of these elements working for you, then they are most certainly working against you!

Chapter 14

Creating Wellness, Not Just Weight Loss

Without doubt, losing weight is one of the most important things that can be done if you are overweight and determined to become super powered. However, you must know that losing weight alone cannot make you a healthy and well person. Weight loss is the issue that seems to get the most attention when it comes to Bio-chemical health. You may think this is a Physical element because it has to do with how your body looks. However, how you lose weight is a Bio-chemical process.

Most weight loss programs, health clubs, books and so on, focus on two elements only: diet and exercise. "Work out and eat right." How many times have you heard that from experts or said it yourself? Of course, it would benefit you if you did those two things, however, this two-sided concept eliminates one of the key elements of success and therefore creates a weak link in your chain. Focusing on all 3 elements is the critical factor in allowing you to sustain your good habits and see them through to consistent healthy life change. By ignoring any single element it does double the damage, first because without an element, that element's benefits are lost and second because without one element, it creates deeper problems that are left over by ignoring it in the first place.

Over the past few years there have been more diet ideas and books than ever before. Many of them contradict each other and complicate things for people who are seeking help.

You may notice this section on weight loss is short compared to the length of many books on the topic. That's because the new science on the topic is much simpler than ever before. The confusion of the past can make it hard to know what type of meal plan to choose going forward. However the wisdom of the past is what will help us cut through the absolute lies that have been told to make some people rich.

While focus on the Bio-chemical element has caused some confusion, it has also done a very good job of putting interest back on how people can help themselves with what they put in their body. I'm also very excited to see that in recent years some very good advice has come out as well. Many of these complicated methods of eating are no longer as popular (thank goodness!) and the school of thought has been simplified by many professionals. This means good news for you!

On the most basic level, when it comes to food, it comes down to calories and basic math. Many experts have now simplified their teachings down to the basic math of weight loss. You have to burn more calories than you take in to lose weight. You have to take in more calories than you burn to gain weight. Calories in and calories out need to be close or even in order to maintain weight. That's it. There's no rocket science or mystery. It is just math. This is what many experts are saying and I agree.

It sounds easy, but do the type of calories or source they come from matter? Great question! To make it fit the SuperHuman lifestyle, the calories you take in must be from as healthy a source as possible. By "as healthy as possible" I mean 80-90 percent of the food and drink you eat should be as natural as possible. Your food ideally would be free of chemicals, preservatives, pesticides, hormones, drugs, and be organic if possible.

Do this to the best of your ability. It can be difficult to have every single thing you eat meet these standards. However, if this is your standard—your super standard—then you will eat food that is closer to these guidelines than if you had lower standards to begin with. For example, and I'll exaggerate here a bit, if you have a choice to eat a snack cake with crème filling sealed in plastic wrap, or a banana, we both know you would want to choose the banana. The banana has healthy calories, is more natural, tastes good, is full of nutrients, etc. A more realistic example is choosing between a hamburger from a fast food joint or making a homemade burger with organic, low fat beef or turkey, natural breads, organic condiments and leafy greens.

Snacks and desserts can be tricky because they can be so small you don't think they count for that much. Beware, they can add up quickly and contain more bad calories than you think. Having self control when it comes to snacks is not something most people would consider a superpower. I'll argue that self-discipline is one of the greatest superpowers that any individual can have.

I believe that self-discipline is difficult for many people. It is, therefore, overlooked, ignored or looked upon as something that will be too difficult to implement in their lives. The superpower of consistency is what I would like you to focus on instead.

Consistency is something you can use to your advantage regularly whether you think so or not. Do you brush your teeth, stop at stop signs, say thank you, or flush the toilet? How about go to the dentist or watch your favorite TV shows? These are all things that you don't have to do or could forget to do, but you don't. Those things may not seem difficult but they are examples of how people who say they can't be consistent are not being honest and recognizing the inner power they already have.

The superpower of consistency is what makes many great leaders great. Consistency is a key part of leadership and as an emerging SuperHuman you could be known as a leader in your community. Therefore developing consistency will be required in order for you to be successful in changing the lives of others.

Live SuperHuman Tool: **Develop consistency by finding one small change that you have wanted to make. Do not pick something hard. Instead, pick something very easy, something that amounts to a 3 percent change rather than a 25 percent change or 50 percent change. For example let's say you have wanted to get up earlier every morning by about 30 minutes so you can have extra time to do any number of healthier things like exercise, eat a better breakfast, or just have more time to spend with your family. Instead of setting your alarm for 30 minutes earlier tomorrow, go to your clock right now and set your alarm for two or three minutes earlier. Then allow yourself to get up three minutes earlier every day for a week. After a week, set your alarm for 3 to 5 minutes earlier again and do the same thing for a week. You can use this 3 percent change method in every aspect of your life in which you want something to be different.**

This book has a number of wonderful tools and tips to help you create habits in your life that will get you to the next level of performance. Believe me, I know full well how difficult consistency can be when it comes to helping someone lose weight and that's why I've have shared my own personal strategies with you in this book. Put them to good use to help you develop the consistent routines that will bring you success. In learning and using what I have shared with you so far, you have already formed a solid foundation. Now you will be able to build on that foundation using guidance and information that can be customized and adjusted to suit your individual needs in your own life.

On a basic level (we will get more advanced as you read on), step one teaches you how you put together a plate of food for a meal. We will start with your large nutrients or proteins, carbohydrates and fats. Proteins are powerful building blocks for muscle, cell walls, energy, and the many tissues and chemicals in your body. Carbs are primarily used for fuel and give you the minute-to-minute energy you need to run your body—particularly your nerve system—and to keep you healthy. Fats are used in many functions and are a very important part of a super meal plan. Fats are used to make up most of your cell walls and nerve system, as well as to make chemicals like hormones. Think about portion size in terms of the size of the palm of your hand. Proteins and carbs should be equal in size, or about as large as your palm (it may be a bit bigger than your palm, like a slice of bread, and that is OK if they are thin enough). Fats should be one-tenth that size, or about the size of the end joint of your thumb. This will give you a 1 to 1 to 1/10 ratio or 1:1:1/10.

When you put together a meal, think of dividing up your plate into thirds that contain the large nutrients. What you are going for is the ratio of protein to carb to fat. One-third of your plate should contain your protein. One third of your plate should contain your carb or carb with fat. A baked potato with butter and sour cream for example. One third should contain your vegetables which are not considered a large nutrient for this purpose because they have such little calorie content with fat, a salad with dressing for example. Remember, when you eat a meal, it should always contain all three. In nature most nutrients are combined together to benefit the recipient. Meats typically have fats and some carbs in them along with the protein. Many vegetables and fruits have carbs and fiber to aid in digestion of the proteins or carbs eaten in the same meal. The biological reason for this is that in nature meals can be scarce and your body needs to get as many of the large nutrients from one source or meal as possible. Proteins slow and moderate the absorption of carbs, which helps prolong your energy. Vegetables help you digest and assimilate the other nutrients along with keeping the digestive tract healthy and clean. The most effective way to eat is to be complete!

Here is an example meal: One-half of a chicken breast seasoned how you like, a small amount of pasta—about a half cup—and a salad with an olive oil based dressing. Literally you could put the chicken and the pasta right next to each other and the rest of the plate could be filled with the salad. To stay in your ratio of 1:1:1/10, your serving sizes of protein and carb should be close to equal and your fat should be very small. Now that you have created a meal that is more in line with your needs, it will be easier for you to get your calories under control while at the same time properly portioning your large nutrients.

The 90 Percent Diet

If I eat well, and within a healthy calorie range 90 percent of the time what do I do with the other 10 percent? I admit right here for everyone to see that I really like to eat some unhealthy foods now and then. Fortunately for me one of the treats I love is chocolate. In addition to curing my craving for something sweet, chocolate has some amazing health benefits. Dark chocolate, unlike milk chocolate, is loaded with antioxidants that help lower your blood pressure. And, of course, antioxidants do many other wonderful things in your body like absorb age causing particles called free radicals (4).

The other unhealthy snack food I like is chips. Chips are on Dr. Mercola's, of mercola.com, list of the top 10 most unhealthy foods along with all other deep fried foods. I mostly avoid chips laden with added coloring, preservatives and MSG. My preference is chips that are as natural as possible and I eat them within my 10 percent range only. The point is that if you want a pastry or a candy bar or a milk shake, that it is OK to eat those things on occasion. Including them in ten percent of your diet would be once every 10 meals, or 100 out of every 1,000 calories (1,000 calories would be about one milkshake).

Here is how I think when I eat in the 10 percent area: I'm not stressed about calories. I'm not stressed about sugar. I'm not stressed about fat, weight gain or even that I'm breaking my own rules and eating less healthy. One of the ways you can ensure your success in eating well is to eat what you want. Just be sure to eat it when you've earned it. Never ever feel bad when you eat within your 10 percent because you've earned it! Eating within your 10 percent is the time for you to reward yourself and to feel good about yourself for the great job you have done.

You can't eat as much as you want and stuff yourself. You must still stay within your 10 percent zone! However, you can eat within your 10 percent zone whenever you want! You can do it at any time of the day or any day during the week. Many meal plans make the mistake of restricting you so much most days and then let you have a "cheat day." That is good except what happens on the cheat day is called a binge. I've heard first-hand testimonials from patients who would eat crazy things on their cheat day like a whole pizza, a tub of ice cream, 4 or 5 hamburgers with fries, soda pop, king sized candy bars, an entire chocolate cake or a combination of all of that. It's crazy!!! Look at what happens to a person's calorie intake who is trying to lose weight. An average serving of ice cream is a half cup and can contain over 150 calories. A one-cup serving of chocolate cake without icing or filling will have approximately 240 calories, and that's a small piece! Imagine eating a pint of ice cream or a whole cake.

Let's do a little math together to see which way is better? Let's say you eat great all week and decide that you are going to have a large brownie and ice cream for your one dessert for the week. And it's your only dessert for the week, which doesn't feel good already because you have been craving some sweets all week. You feel good about yourself because you haven't let yourself give into a craving so you'll have just a little more than normal. After all, you've been so good it won't hurt, right? So you have a large brownie and a bowl of ice cream. Even a small bowl is more than half a cup so we'll say you have about a cup of ice cream or two medium scoops. Total calories: about 600 to 800! I hope you were eating strictly within your 90/10 zone because that eats up nearly all of your 10 percent, at 7.6 percent, for the week! Yikes, and you had to suffer all week to get there. In calories eating 1700 calories a day gives you 11,900 calories a week, of which your 10 percent zone is 1190.

If you do that four times every month, that's 3,000 to 4,000 extra calories per month! Are you likely to succeed for very long dragging yourself thought that torture every week? Heck no, not with busy daily routines that force you to grab something on the go between running to work, social get togethers, dropping the kids at school, dance, football, cheer, and so on. That is why so many people suffer with diet problems. It is not easy to stick with healthy eating when you do it that way. It's not even easy for me and I am already in habit of doing what we are talking about.

Live SuperHuman Tool: **To lose weight you must burn more calories than you consume. Period. The healthier the calories, the healthier and lighter you will be! You are what you eat as they say ... so don't eat junk! You are too good for that. Treat your body as a temple, a spiritual place where only good things are allowed in.**

The emotional stress of forcing yourself to go back to eating well while knowing it is going to be a while before you can have another snack is harder in real life than in theory. I also want to point out that we are only talking about one single dessert in this example. This example does not include eating any other high calorie food like pizza, pop, milk shakes, fries, burgers, etc., and that makes this example extremely conservative.

Let's look at this the SuperHuman way. You eat within your 90 percent for all your major meals for an entire month. Averaging four meals per day, or about 108 well balanced meals using the 1:1:1/10 calorie ratio system (or using the Nutritional Typing personalized for you, which you'll learn about in an upcoming chapter), you'll have room in the month for about 10 to 15 meals that are in your 10 percent. Then you can have a meal that is not within your ideal plan every two to three days! Anyone, SuperHuman or not, can do that! This gives you the room in your everyday life to be a realistic person and never have to beat yourself up.

Let's keep going. Let's say you eat nine meals in the month that are in your 10 percent zone. That means that you still have some room to wiggle for other cravings that might pop up. When you can satisfy a craving you won't want or need to binge, or even eat too much to satisfy your appetite for it.

Live SuperHuman Dessert Secret:

Here is how you do it: you just have a piece or two of dark chocolate, or a few peanut m&m's, when you have your cravings. A piece of dark chocolate the size of a Hershey's Kiss has only 20 calories. If you had one piece every day that would only equal about 600 calories for the month. If you had 5 peanut m&m's that would have about 45 calories. If you had half a Fun Size pack of m&m's at a time and went through 2 packs per week, that would total about only 720 calories. Eating a small brownie or snack size Butterfinger or Snickers candy bar, that have about 100 calories, two times per week still puts you in at only 800 calories for the month. Compare that to an extra 3000-4000 calories in the cake and bowl of ice cream dessert we talked about before. If you don't like chocolate, apply the same to what you like.

Let's just say that I'm wrong, (but if you do the math for yourself, you will find this information to be very accurate). But let's pretend I'm wrong by 50 percent and you ate half as much for dessert on a binge and double the smaller snacks. You would still come out over 1500-2000 more than you would if you satisfied those little cravings regularly as I suggest. Less calories = less weight!

Chapter 15

How Do I Eat?

I WANT TO LIVE SUPERHUMAN...HOW DO I EAT?

So, how do SuperHumans eat? Among professionals I have worked and consulted with, it is unanimously agreed upon that metabolic typing, or Nutritional Typing™, is the very best way to eat. Nutritional Typing™ is the mother of all diets. If you were to visualize all types of diets—blood typing, high carb, low carb, no carb, eating in zones, or high protein as branches on a family tree, then Nutritional or metabolic typing would be the trunk and roots of the tree from which all others grew. For example, blood type eating is one small part of Nutritional Typing™. An excellent book on this subject is called The Metabolic Typing Diet by inventor and developer of metabolic typing William Wolcott. His work is fascinating and genius to say the very least. This book can teach you to eat in a way that matches your body's specific needs and enhances how your body utilizes foods to get SuperHuman benefits. Two of the world's top leaders in wellness have come together to provide resources to help you learn your Nutritional Type™: Dr. Joe Mercola with his Nutritional Typing™ and Dr. Patrick Gentempo with the Creating Wellness System. Gentempo's program shows you how to take a calorie-based diet (like the 1:1:1/10 ratio system on page 58) and take it up to the next level with metabolic typing.

These programs simply customize eating to you, and I'm a huge fan of customizing your choices to your own personal needs! When I say "customizing," I don't just mean what's "good for you," "tastes good to you," or "healthy for you." While these programs are all of that, true diet customizing takes into account things that we don't typically think about—like our thousands of years of heritage, what our genes are made of, which cultures my body prefers foods from and so on. What you must realize is that the world has become so small that you can get almost any kind of food you want at any time you want it. This is great when it comes to eating because it allows you eat what your body was designed to eat.

Here is a brief overview of how Nutritional Typing™ can help you Live SuperHuman. It would seem silly for someone who has Japanese and Polynesian Island heritage to eat only foods that are grown in the mid-western United States, like corn, wheat grains, beef, etc., simply because that is where they currently live. Because of genetic evolution, people have metabolic types that more efficiently use certain kinds of food. Someone of Japanese and Polynesian descent, for example, needs lots of fish, rice grains, small game and exotic fruits to more closely match the kind of food their genes have evolved to tolerate, or the kind of food that's appropriate for their metabolic type. The same would go for people from the northern Mediterranean coastal region. People with Greek and Italian heritage have metabolic types that do very well with olive oils, breads, fish, and pastas from the region. If your metabolic type does better with one type of food than another, eating food that is incompatible with your metabolic type could result in weight gain, loss of energy, lower your immune function, and digestive problems disease.

Don't be overwhelmed. It is extremely easy to eat for your metabolic type if you follow the guidelines in the book The Metabolic Typing Diet. It's even easier if you get guidance through LiveSuperHuman.com. Nutritional Typing™ turns eating into a healing part of your life and much more closely matches your body's specific needs when it comes to your biochemistry. A very important benefit of metabolic typing is that foods that are right for your metabolic type have healing properties for your body. The more you eat foods that match your metabolic needs the stronger and healthier you become. You can reverse disease processes, gain strength and energy, and simply improve your general wellness by eating according to what your body was genetically engineered to digest and use.

Live SuperHuman Tool: **Nutritional Typing is recognized as one of the very best ways to eat your food. Find out your Nutritional Type today!**

Conversely, if you repeatedly eat foods that are not right for your biochemistry and metabolic type, you will weaken your body. Over years of metabolizing nutrients that aren't right for you, your entire body suffers the consequences. Some people feel the effects more than others, but we all want to be SuperHuman, having spectacular health and vitality, not just being alive with mediocre health. To achieve that goal, regardless of how you think your food makes you feel, how you eat matters a great deal.

I understand there are dozens of ways to eat out there and these are only two examples. The goal here is to educate you on a real world solution that works; a solution like Nutritional Typing that gets you to a place where you can eat as your body is designed for.

Physical
Bio-chemical
Neuro-spiritual

Chapter 16

Do SuperHumans Take Nutritional Supplements?

Supplements have been a topic of debate for years. Some experts say you should get your nutrients from food (which I would agree with—you should), and that you should not need to take vitamins if you are eating healthy. Others say supplements are a must. What's a SuperHuman to do? Let me break this down for you so that there are no questions in your mind regarding this topic ever again.

When I say I agree that you should be able to get your nutrients from food I mean it. It makes sense and it certainly simplifies things. After all, people have been doing it for thousands of years. However, this is not the whole story, nor is it the whole truth. When considering the issue of getting nutrition from food or from supplements you must remember that we live in a free market, capitalist world when it comes to food. Food is a multi-trillion dollar industry worldwide. In order for farmers to make a living in this competitive industry, a couple things have to happen.

First, farmers have to be business people. They have families to feed and employees to pay. This means they have to make business decisions that don't always align with growing the food in a way that ensures that as many nutrients as possible end up in the food. For example, soils that get used over and over again year after year to grow crops become nutrient deficient over time as all those nutrients are sucked up by the growing plants. In order to replenish the soils properly farmers would need to till very deeply to churn up new nutrients. To till soils deeper means different, more advanced and powerful equipment has to be used, which costs lots of money. Soils could also be replenished by adding nutrients back into the soils, rather than just using fertilizers to grow the plants, which costs lots of money. There are other growing methods but either way it comes down to a business decision, and a business owner has to feed his own family, which means costs have to be kept down whenever possible. Ironically, you'd think they would want to feed their family healthy, nutrient rich foods.

Small organic operations are doing a better job of producing healthier, organically grown crops. Even though locally grown foods are better because they are likely coated with less to no poisons and may have higher nutrient contents your selection of foods will be limited to what grows well in your area seasonally. I would say that you should buy whatever organic meats and veggies you can from your local producers. Just know that if you only eat locally, you will be getting a fraction of the total micro nutrients like phyto-nutrients, flavinoids and antioxidants you likely need for optimal health. Food contains thousands of tiny nutrients that contribute to your overall wellness and disease ability fighting other than the commonly known vitamins and minerals. To get the most of these, you should eat a varied selection of food, which may be difficult to do from strictly local foods in your microclimate especially for your Nutrition Type.

The second thing that happens in the food industry, as in every industry, is technological advancement. In food, that means everything from better machinery, to growing foods hydroponically (in water) rather than in soil. Genetically modified foods (GMOs) are another thing technology has provided, though personally I don't consider GMOs an advancement in terms of wellness because consuming GMO foods can take you in the wrong direction on the scale between health and illness. Regardless of the change, advancing technology is expensive.

The bottom line to you and me is that our foods don't have the quantity of nutrients they used to have in them even 50 years ago. Here is a point that blows my mind and should answer any debate on this topic for most people. If you were to eat an average size bowl of salad (say 2 cups) in 1950, that 2 cups of salad would have a certain amount of vitamins, minerals, and nutrients inside it. If you were to eat the same 2-cup bowl of salad today, how many bowls do you think you would have to eat to get the same amount of vitamins, minerals and nutrients that you could get back in 1950? I have asked this question to hundreds of people and I get a lot of great guesses like, double, triple or even 10 times the amount. Imagine 10 bowls of salad. That's not even close! The answer is that you would have to eat over 23 bowls of salad—nearly 50 cups to get the same amount of nutrients today that you could have gotten 60 years ago in only 2 cups. Today, people simply can't eat the massive quantities of food required to feed your body all of the nutrients it needs. Now tell me, should you eat 23 bowls of salad or do you think you should take supplements—in addition to eating well—to help get you the right nutrition? If you don't take top quality supplements then your body simply doesn't have the fuel it needs to live anywhere near SuperHuman.

Let's get back to something I said earlier about getting your nutrients from food. It is true that your body absorbs nutrients more readily and easily from foods than it does from supplements that have isolated nutrients like multi-vitamins. That is why you see huge nutrient amounts listed on the labels of supplement bottles. That is also why the pills from the world's best vitamin companies have become so big and you need to take so many of them. The size and quantity of tablets you must take is a complaint I hear from patients all the time. A literal overload of isolated vitamins has to be put into a supplement in order to give your body a chance to absorb the portion it needs. Another huge problem (and waste of your money) is that the supplement industry is a business just like farming. To get top quality, natural, nutrient combinations and to get enough of them packed in to a pill can be expensive. In addition to expense, many supplements can actually be worse for you because the nutrients in them are synthetic or derived from sources that are toxic, rather than sourced from all natural, organic, non-genetically modified, toxin-free sources, because it is cheaper.

Lyle MacWilliam and the company NutriSearch have published a book called *The Comparative Guide to Nutritional Supplements* for over half a decade. NutriSearch independently tests nearly every nutritional supplement on the market. Last year that number was over 1500 different multi-vitamins and minerals. Only multi-vitamins are tested and then ranked on a 5-star rating system. The ratings are based on 18 different criteria, such as antioxidant strength, potency and bioavailability of vitamin E, liver health, bone health, eye health, etc. This testing has led to the creation of the world's leading authority and trusted source on vitamins. In other words, NutriSearch's book will tell you exactly which supplements are worth your money.

I get people everyday in my office who tell me they are taking a variety of supplements: calcium, antioxidants, vitamin C, juices, joint formulas, cleanses, vitamin D, B-complex, and on and on. They also tell me how much they spend every month. Are you ready for this? Some of them spend upwards of $300 per month! That's crazy and often, it's a complete waste of money because they haven't spent time determining which of those supplements they should take.

In my office, I don't even recommend — let alone sell — vitamins that are not top rated in the Comparative Guide or that don't use cutting-edge technology to ensure your body gets **food based nutrients** rather than chemically isolated nutrients, which it cannot easily absorb. The top rated supplements receive what is called a 5-star Gold award for quality. I don't want you wasting your money and energy taking supplements that don't provide enough value for you to take. I want you to stop wasting your money! So here's my advice: get the best vitamins there are...this is your life! Many products that rate at less than 2 stars cost 2 to 3 times what the top rated vitamins cost. I have researched all this information and am happy to pass along the results to you here, and more at the extension of this book LiveSuperHuman.com! However, if you need to see for yourself, I recommend you get a *Comparative Guide* and see where your vitamin ranks.

Physical
Bio-chemical
Neuro-spiritual

Chapter 17

GAP

In Chapter 10 we discussed the nerve system and how it controls and coordinates the whole body. The primary job of the brain and nerve system is to expand your General Adaptive Potential or GAP. This is explained well by patient communication expert Dr. David Fletcher and his term, GAP, will help you understand the great importance of a healthy, disturbance-free nerve system. Literally the less disturbance you have in your nerve system, the greater your GAP!

A greater GAP equals better adaptation and fewer illnesses for you. The year 2008 was a landmark year for diseases worldwide. Historically, infectious diseases, such as tuberculosis, AIDS, and Malaria were leading causes of death globally. In 2008, for the first time in history, lifestyle diseases such as heart disease, became the cause of death for more people than infectious diseases. These figures are a nightmare for the planet. It seems as though people have less and less GAP. I'm telling you now that my mission is to reverse this statistic before the year 2020 by helping people become so healthy that they won't have to deal with any of these problems. Greater GAP equals greater wellness.

What do the leading causes of death have to do with your GAP and your Bio-chemical health? It tells you exactly what supplements to take to help expand your GAP and avoid negative health issues. For example, if heart disease and cancer are two leading causes of death, then we need to take supplements and live in a way that strengthens us, making us less susceptible to those diseases. I'm giving you that information at your fingertips. Information that will help you learn to change your destiny, expand your GAP and a live longer, better life.

Here is a way to understand how the central nervous system is related to your GAP. Imagine a hypothetical situation of two children, one child who was subluxated, or has nerve disturbance, from a difficult birth and can't adapt well to the environment. This child might have trouble learning things, may develop slowly, and may be less able to learn from mistakes and then change behavior, and so on. Does this sound like a child that will grow into a healthy, vibrant adult? Or does this sound like a child that may have disabilities, behavior problems, and physical limitations? The second child had its nerve system checked at birth or very young, and has no nerve disturbance or subluxation. This child can learn quickly, and mentally and physically develops at a rapid rate. This child learns from mistakes, develops a strong immune system, and constantly does new and more challenging things.

Which of these children has a greater ability to adapt or a greater GAP? Silly question, I know. Which of these children has more potential to achieve greatness that contributes to society in life and not just exist? Which of these children has a greater capacity to contribute to the world in meaningful ways? What I'm talking about here is the future of the world, a future in which people can contribute and give back to society, rather than suck off society for free handouts or whatever scraps they can muster. That isn't life!

These examples don't describe everyone and aren't meant to force anyone into any particular corner. The point should not be missed that the odds can be stacked against you or for you. Just think of how many people, to varying degrees, have a GAP that is closed down or has been in the process of closing for their entire life. Life is about expansion and growth. Almost everything grows, by the way, which makes growth one of the most natural phenomenon on the planet! Trees grow, grass grows, people grow, rivers grow, knowledge and consciousness grow and grow. Your GAP naturally wants to grow as well.

The greater adaptability you have, the more SuperHuman you can become. The greater adaptability you have, the more likely you are to resist disease and illness. The greater adaptability you have, the more likely you are to live an active and healthy life to 100 years old or more.

Knowing and being able to teach you what supplements to take to expand your GAP comes from over a decade of research and data accumulation. I can tell you with absolute certainty that what goes into your body determines what you will get out of your body. Put great stuff in so you get great stuff out. You see, great nutrition isn't only about treating dis-ease, it is about making your body so healthy that you don't get dis-eased in the first place. That is the essence of wellness.

Live SuperHuman Tool: **Expand your GAP with powerful supplements and regular chiropractic care to remove subluxations.**

The leading causes of death teach us that we want to take supplements - like we discussed in chapter 16 - that provide us protection from 1. medicine 2. cancer and 3. heart disease and most importantly help us live a life full of greater vitality and wellness. Well, if you don't get sick and don't need medicine then you take care of number one.

Physical
Bio-chemical
Neuro-spiritual

Chapter 18

Drinking Milk Can Make You Fat

Drinking Milk Can Make You Fat

I saw an ad that says if I eat dairy products it will help me lose weight. Is that true? Let's get right down to it and dispel this **myth** now. The claim that milk can help you lose weight amazes me and is proof of how statistics and fine print can be twisted to benefit interested parties. The three-a-day ad campaign was created based on a research study that found people who eat a diet that includes at least three diary products per day weigh less, on average, than people who don't.

Claims that low-fat dairy products or calcium can help people lose weight could be totally false! Dairy products and/or calcium intake do not promote weight loss according to Dr. Amy Lanou. "Don't believe the hype," says Dr. Lanou, assistant professor in the department of health and wellness at the University of North Carolina in Asheville. "The ads that promote milk as helping to achieve a healthy weight are misleading; the science does not support these ads."

Lanou, and Neal D. Barnard with the Physicians Committee for Responsible Medicine in Washington, DC, evaluated evidence from 49 clinical trials that assessed whether dairy products or calcium can help people lose weight.

Out of 49 clinical trials, 41 showed no effects of diary or calcium on weight, two showed an increase in body weight with a dairy regimen, and one showed a lower rate of weight gain. Only five showed weight loss occurred. Only five out of 49 trials!

"Our findings demonstrate that increasing dairy product intake does not consistently result in weight or fat loss and may actually have the opposite effect," Lanou and Barnard concluded and published in Nutrition Reviews in 2008.

In order to clarify some of your thoughts over dairy products I'd like share more about them. Much of this information comes from financial and wellness expert Professor Paul Zane Pilzer and his book The Wellness Revolution, which I highly recommend you read. There are a couple questions I'd like you to think about as you read this:

The political lobby of the American Dairy Association is extremely strong. Is the ADA's legislative pull really being used to promote true wellness in American kids and adults?

If this upcoming information is even half true, what are the negative health effects on people who follow these ad campaigns' advice?

Milk producers treat their dairy cattle with recombinant bovine growth hormone (rBGH) to boost milk production. But rBGH also increases udder infections, according to Samuel S. Epstein, MD, Chairman of the Cancer Prevention Coalition. Dr. Epstein states, "Hormonal milk is often contaminated with pus cells, resulting from mastitis in cows due to hyperstimulation of milk production, and also with antibiotics used to treat the mastitis. Other abnormalities include increased fatty acids, which are incriminated in heart disease (5).

Martin Donohoe, MD, and Rick North, Science Advisor and Project Director, respectively, for the Oregon Physicians for Social Responsibility Campaign for Safe Food, state about rGBH: "It is well known that rBGH increases levels of another growth hormone, IGF-1, which is identical in cows and humans. At elevated levels, IGF-1 is known to increase cancer rates in humans" (6). Dr. Epstein is adamant: "More serious are major risks of breast, colon, and prostate cancers due to increased IGF levels in hormonal milk. Evidence for this has been documented in about 50 scientific publications over the past three decades." (5)

Milk and milk by-products are leading the charge to make it more difficult for people to lose weight and create wellness. Milk has been linked to many conditions such as allergies, gas, constipation, obesity, cancer, heart disease, infectious diseases, and osteoporosis. Osteoporosis? But wait, you thought milk had calcium that fights osteoporosis, right?

Several studies show that drinking milk may cause rather than prevent osteoporosis. This happens because the nutrients in milk are designed to build 1500 pound animals, not 150 pound people. The proteins in milk, called casein, and its pH, require your body to leach calcium from your own bones in order to balance your pH during digestion. These large proteins also make it difficult for your body to absorb calcium from milk. Calcium contained naturally in vegetables, or whole food supplements is much healthier, easier to absorb, and more abundant. One cup of calcium-enriched orange juice contains more calcium than fortified milk at 350 milligrams compared to 302 milligrams in a cup of milk.

According to North, milk can be loaded with growth hormones and antibiotics as well as carry infectious diseases, like bovine spongiform encephalopathy or Mad Cow Disease. An average cow can naturally produce up to 10 pounds of milk in a single day. Dairy farm cows are made to produce up to 10 times that amount at 100 pounds of milk per day. This is made possible because dairy cows are given massive amounts of hormones designed to increase milk production. This often makes their udders so large they drag on the ground resulting in recurrent infection and requiring constant antibiotics. The USDA allows milk to contain from 1 to 1.5 million white blood cells per milliliter. White blood cells are what kill off infection and are what we call pus when near a wound.

How healthy do you think it is for kids to drink hormones, antibiotics, and pus that remain in the milk after processing? What, if any, do you think the health consequences could be?

In the book The Wellness Revolution, Pilzer states that hormones used in milk, BGH, have been connected to increasing the average breast size of teenage human girls and decreasing the age of the onset of menses. Additionally, growth hormones are a known factor in causing malignant tumors in the human breast and other tissues. Numerous consumer groups have insisted milk containing these hormones be banned or at least labeled properly with a warning but sadly the FDA turns a blind eye to the issue.

Large scale milk production is disgusting and bad for the environment and the cows. A dairy cow may produce 100 pounds of milk, but it also produces 120 pounds of waste each day. That is equal to the amount of waste 24 people would produce and none of that waste is given sewage treatment. Each cow consumes 81 pounds of grains and vegetables, plus 45 gallons of water per day! Although natural cows may live 20 to 25 years, cows in dairy production sadly live only four to five years because they burn out from the hormones and constant artificial pregnancies (induced to keep up the population of milk producing cows on the farm) that turn them from living creatures into grotesque milking machines according to Pilzer.

Pilzer states "The worst thing about dairy products is not the disease they cause or the torture of the animals but that it is a major contributor to more than 61 percent of our population being overweight and obese."

Americans eat about four pounds of food per day, and nearly 40 percent of that is from milk and dairy products. With such a high percentage of food from dairy, it must be healthy you would think. Think again...**Milk contains:**

- **Zero fiber, and is filled with saturated fat and cholesterol, one glass is 49 percent fat.**
- **Cheeses are more than 65 percent fat.**
- **One 12-ounce glass contains as much saturated fat as eight strips of bacon.**
- **A 12-ounce glass of beer only contains 144 calories and zero fat. A 12-ounce glass of milk contains 300 calories and 16 grams of fat.**

- **Four tablespoons of half-and-half added to a cup of coffee contains 80 percent of the saturated fat you should consume in an entire day at 15 grams.**

Pilzer states: "to counter the undisputed truth of these facts, the dairy industry came up with the deception of '2 percent' and 'low-fat' milk. In reality, 2 percent milk contains 24 to 33 percent calories from fat and is only slightly less fattening than whole milk which contains 3 percent fat by weight. Milk producers even went as far as to label cottage cheese as 'low-fat,' which contains 20 percent calories of fat. This prompted the FDA to order diary producers to stop promoting milk products as low or nonfat foods."

How did we get to where we are today with such a high percentage of our diets as dairy products? Innovative entrepreneurs figured out ways to produce milk at low prices, then used their profits to build self-perpetuating marketing—a political organization now known as the ADA.

The ADA lobbied the federal government to subsidize overproduction of what is now nearly an 8 billion dollar a year industry, and then forced milk into the diets of children through mandatory school lunch programs. Most adult humans of every race are lactose intolerant. Caucasians, who comprise most of the milk market, have sadly learned to accept the accompanying allergic reactions, heartburn, upset stomach, diarrhea, gas, and diabetes as a part of everyday life, explains Pilzer.

You cannot treat these symptoms with medication. It takes a SuperHuman lifestyle to get to the root cause of these issues and heal yourself with your natural healing ability.

My kids know to stay clear of cow milk at school and in general. My son and daughter have grown up on alternatives, and to this day one of my son's favorite drinks is rice milk.

Live SuperHuman Tool: **Stay away from milk that is not 100 percent organic and raw. Sheep milk is best, then goat, and finally cow milk. Very few states allow raw milk to be produced and sold legally. Alternatives are rice and soy. Recent studies advise avoiding soy consumption in large amounts because it has estrogen hormone mimicking properties. Rice, however, does not have high nutrient value but is inexpensive and usually organic.**

Local milk and beef producers are gaining major popularity all over the country. Small farms are doing an incredible job of raising 100 percent organic livestock that are loved and genuinely cared for. Organic meats and dairy products that are raised in your local area help you avoid all of the nasty issues mentioned earlier and are a great solution for you to be healthier.

Chapter 19

A New Cure for Cancer: Theory or Reality?

What Causes Cancer?

In addition to discussing what cancer is in this section, I'm going to tell you about forward thinking cancer treatment technologies...It is up to you, and even worthwhile to consult a physician, to determine if these types are right for you. I want you to stop, open your mind, and understand that these ideas are gaining traction in some arenas while being violently attacked in others.

I will tell you now that when you get down to the very root of it, cancer is caused by one thing: stress. That stress may be Physical, Bio-Chemical or Neuro-Spiritual (also referred to as mental or psychological). Many disease experts argue that all disease is caused by stress at its root. A minor portion of disease is genetically caused but that is rarely the primary issue. Only about 5 percent of the population worldwide is born with genetic defects. That means that 95 percent of world's population has nearly optimal gene expression at birth, says cellular biologist and author of The Biology of Belief, Dr. Bruce Lipton.

Dr. Lipton purports that genetics have relatively little sway over a person's health, making the case that health is only influenced about 30 percent by genetics. That means the vast majority of what happens to your health is related to your environment, lifestyle, and perceptions—in other words, stresses.

The problem with stress in any of its three forms, Physical, Bio-Chemical, or Neuro-Spiritual, is that it has an accumulative effect on the body. Your nervous system constantly adapts your body but it can only do so much to fight off stress. Ultimately, when the cumulative damage is too much, disease is the result.

Cancer is thought by many to be a lifestyle stress disease and there will never be an ultimate "cure for cancer" until the lifestyle stress is addressed on an individual basis. You may not like to hear that but that is largely how the body works and why there are so many testimonials of people who changed their lifestyle after being diagnosed with cancer and healed themselves. The body can only adapt so much and that is why some people don't heal even if they change their lifestyle. I feel that all-or-none beliefs about the cause of cancer don't account for all we don't understand in the universe and cancer can rarely happen even if you do things right. The point is to do everything you can now, in advance, to avoid a battle with cancer.

Miracles occur, as well, and in my opinion should not be discounted. I tell my patients that whether you heal in six days or two years, it really doesn't matter. A miracle is a miracle, especially if you thought it would never get better. I have a dear friend who had abnormal blood tests that led to an MRI of his liver. The MRI showed a tumor or mass, that was 3 centimeters in diameter. Essentially what that means is that you have fatal liver cancer and are going to die in three to six months. A few days later he told me that he felt a small "pop" in his liver and heard a voice tell him he "was healed" while he was alone at home one night. Trust me, this is not the kind of person who hears voices. This is a self-made, powerful business man who is used to telling people what to do and getting his way. He goes to church sometimes but would not be considered overly religious or even spiritual by any means. After speaking with his wife and beginning to prepare arrangements for his death a couple days later again he heard in his head, "I told you, you're fine." At his next doctor visit about a week later they did another, more detailed imaging scan, a CT scan, to verify details of the tumor but the there was no longer a tumor, or any abnormality to be found! The astonished doctors told him to count his lucky stars because it was a miracle.

That is a true miracle, but what if you have cancer now? How would you treat it to live long enough and vitally enough to get to the root solution and address the stress? Only when you clean up the underlying cause will the cure be found. Below is a potential answer to solving the problem long enough to find your ultimate cure.

An Italian oncologist, Dr. Tullio Simoncini, and others like cancer researcher Dr. Ralph Moss and pH expert Dr. Robert O. Young have done research that has led them to conclude that something as simple as a fungus, Candida, is not only a leading cause of cancer but perhaps that cancer itself could be a fungus. What we call a tumor, may be nothing more than your body's attempt at protecting itself from that fungus. Unbelievable? Read on…

Dr. Simoncini claims to have been able to link cancer to fungus in several studies, showing between 79 to 97 percent of all cancer patients also have Candida Systemic. Candida, the way I refer to it here and the way it is referred to in alternative medicine, is unassociated with its use in clinical medicine to refer to the fungus that causes vaginal yeast infections or thrush.

He isn't the only one making these conclusions. Dr. Ralph Moss at the University of Arizona has been researching sodium bicarbonate, or baking soda, as a cancer treatment over the last decade. Dr. Moss' research, completed in 2009, has been found to enhance anti-tumor activity, increase tumor pH, and inhibit spontaneous metastasis, or spreading, in a cancerous condition.

Mark Sircus, the director of the International Medical Veritas Association (IMVA) and author of Winning the War on Cancer states that "all cancer sufferers should keep in mind that pH is the regulatory authority that controls most cellular processes. The pH balance of the human bloodstream is recognized by medical physiology texts as one of the most important biochemical balances in all of human body chemistry."

Sodium bicarbonate, or baking soda, is a potent anti-fungal substance. The problem with anti-fungal drugs, however, is that fungi—as innately intelligent critters—are extremely resilient and can adapt to a new environment in three to four days. Anti-fungal drugs are very ineffective. Fungi have survived for millions of years through ice ages, floods, volcanic eruptions and so on. How is a drug going to have an impact on the life of a fungus? The fungi do not adapt to baking soda when it is applied as a treatment directly to the cancer or tumor, unlike systemic drug treatments like antifungal medications. Sodium bicarbonate prevents the fungi from adapting because it changes the pH from acid to alkaline so quickly.

Dr. Sircus says the ideal way to utilize sodium bicarbonate is in a heated combination with 100 percent pure maple syrup. This combination was discovered by controversial folk healer Jim Kelmun who amazingly claims that this simple home remedy can stop and reverse the deadly growth of cancers.

Eating sugar is contrary to most health logic in treating illness. Cancer cells consume about 15 times the glucose sugars than that of normal cells. Thus when sodium bicarbonate is fused with the maple syrup the cancer cells gobble it up rapidly alkalizing their own pH. The actual recommended formula is to mix one part baking soda with three parts 100 percent pure maple syrup in a small saucepan. Stir briskly and heat the mixture for 5 minutes. On Cancer Tutor, an online guide to alternative cancer treatments, the Jim Kelmun protocol recommends taking 1 teaspoon per day, but you could probably do this several times a day.

The Arizona Cancer Center researchers have shown how manipulation of tumor pH with sodium bicarbonate enhances some forms of chemotherapy (8).

Remember, our Source or God's intelligent design is in all things, including fungi. Candida colonies are highly communicative with one another just like human communities. It makes sense to attack the tumor site directly with Dr. Simoncini's method and raise system wide pH with oral maple syrup mix.

Why the Baking Soda Cancer Cure is Not Available Everywhere

Unfortunately, doctors like, Moss, Young, Sircus and Simoncini are yet another example of revolutionary thinkers who's simple genius and innovative ideas have the ability to shut down the medical cancer fighting industry. I don't know the reason that ideas like these are shunned, however, I do know that if cancer goes away, a multi -billion dollar industry of doctors, scientists, hospitals, treatment centers, foundations and drug companies all go out of business. I do believe that the people treating an individual with cancer want to help and find a cure. Ironically, the disease is what keeps them fighting the fight and, in fact, there is an industry that is sustained by the disease's existence.

Preventive Measures for Candida with Lifestyle

If the cause of some cancer is the Candida fungus, then we need to address the root cause of the fungi. How can you tell if you have Candida in your body, which might eventually lead to cancer?

According to Dr. Mercola, a good sign that Candida is on the loose is feeling "run down" and developing a craving for sugars and carbohydrates, as this is the main fuel for the growing amounts of yeast in your intestine. The more sugar and grains you eat, the more the yeast grows out of control. Eventually, this will weaken your immune system, which in turn can allow it to infiltrate various other organs.

An imbalance in intestinal flora can also lead to other more common and less lethal health problems such as:

- Vaginitis
- Irritable bowel syndrome
- Weight gain
- Food allergies
- Migraines
- Asthma
- Depression
- Chronic fatigue syndrome and fibromyalgia

Yogurt can be a terrible way to balance your intestinal flora, contrary to what many people think. Most yogurt is full of sugar and is usually made from dairy products from non-organic sources. Additionally the concentration of probiotics in yogurt is nowhere near what you can get from proper supplementation. Everyday my kids and I take a special formula I call my SuperHuman Drink that contains an exceptional balance of healthy pro and prebiotics to help with this delicate balance.

There are 79 different toxins released into the blood stream by the metabolism and die-off of Candida. This is why people with yeast overgrowth often feel bad. Two of these toxins, alcohol and acetaldehyde, which causes hangovers, are in such high amounts in people with chronic yeast problems that they can actually feel drunk.

Acetaldehyde also reacts with the neurotransmitter dopamine, the "feel good hormone," which is why people with fungal overgrowth often experience mental and emotional stresses such as anxiety, depression, poor concentration, and feeling spaced-out.

What makes sense to me about the fungus-cancer theory is that the lifestyle that prevents the growth of fungus is the same lifestyle that is lived by the population of people who rarely get cancer. Coincidence? Not a chance! Live SuperHuman and you are making your way there already!

Live SuperHuman Tool: **Science estimates the human body averages over 10,000 potential opportunities to develop cancer per day! Lowering your risk of cancer is a superpower you naturally have by being strong and healthy. Strengthen this power through improving Bio-chemical & Neuro-spiritual health.**

Physical
Bio-chemical
Neuro-spiritual

Chapter 20

Bad Medicine

In our first conversation, my patient Julie tells me that at the ripe old age of 21 years old she can't remember a day she hasn't had a headache. At the age of 12 she recalls telling her dad that her head hurt and he asked her if that happened often. She replied, "my head always hurts, doesn't yours?" By the age of 16 Julie had seen almost every specialist including neurologists, pain specialists, OBgyn's, hormone specialists, therapists, and her medical doctor ... which is how she ended up on Paxil for severe migraine headaches.

Off label prescribing, when a drug is given to a person to treat a condition the drug is not meant to treat, is becoming more common in medicine. Unfortunately for Julie the drug covered up her symptoms for almost five years. She went from severe headaches, which she rated an 8 out of 10, and migraines that incapacitated her three to four times a week to zero headaches for a couple years. But eventually, the medicine was unable to cover up Julie's headaches. When she arrived at my office, she was having three migraines a week again.

While the drug did make her feel better temporarily, it also stopped the family's search for a real cure, and ultimately, for the cause of the problem. All the while Julie's decaying spine and subluxated (remember: nerve disturbance caused by stress) nerve system continued to wreak havoc on her body. Her endocrine system began to malfunction and she began to have severe hormone imbalances. She could not have a comfortable or regular menstrual cycle. Her body began to metabolize food into fat at an alarming rate, and she entered my office over 100 pounds overweight.

The poor kid, was all I could think at the time. To treat a simple problem, she was on a drug that causes anxiety, depression and suicidal thoughts and it caused her to gain wait and deal with the devastating effect that has on one's self-esteem. After an exam, nerve scans and x-rays it was clear to me that no other doctor had even tried to locate the cause of her problem, which likely occurred at birth.

Even worse, the doctor who gave her the drug actually thought he did her a favor. Migraines don't even make the list for off-label uses for Paxil. Paxil is contraindicated in all patients under 18, meaning it should not be prescribed to patients under 18. In the United States, the FDA requires the drug to carry a black box warning, which is its "most serious type of warning in prescription drug labeling," due to increased risk of suicidal behavior. Ironically, one of the side effects for Paxil is headache.

Remember, your body performs over 6 trillion chemical reactions every second. Every chemical reaction depends upon and is coordinated around every other chemical reaction in the body. All of this is governed and monitored by your brain and nervous system. It is reckless and unconscionable to me to think that you can put a strong, manmade, disruptive chemical into the body without considering the possible negative effects. The type of doctoring Julie received needs to stop.

Left to fend for herself at 21 years old and trying to find her own solution to her health problems, Julie ended up in my office. I'm filled with gratitude that her aunt told her about me. I told her the truth about how the body is self-healing and the nervous system coordinates those healing processes.

Can you imagine being stuck in a body that has malfunctioned since birth in such a way that you are in constant pain? Can you imagine what your perception of the world would be? Can you imagine what your potential would have been? Can you imagine what your potential would be once you are healed? Can you imagine what it would be like to have a life free from that kind of suffering? After getting off the drugs and under chiropractic care ... Julie can.

Unfortunately Julie's story is not uncommon and Julie is only one of hundreds of patients like this I have seen in my small practice. She is one of millions of people who have the same type of story. As a SuperHuman I am calling you now to share what you know with anyone who is suffering. All you have to do is share some of the valuable information in this book, and you could be responsible for saving a life. This is not a privilege or an "I will if I feel like it" type of thing. This is an obligation that we as SuperHumans have to humanity. We actually have the superpower to save lives. So go out and use this power to your full potential! Don't just do it by words, lead by example.

Chapter 21

Why can drugs be so bad?

Remember the code. Rule 1: always maximize your powers, never give them up!
Misusing antibiotics can lead to the development of deadly strains of bacteria that are resistant to drugs and cause more than 88,000 deaths due to hospital-acquired infections. NSAIDs or non steroidal anti-inflammatories like aspirin or naproxen, have been identified as the causing of up to 20,000 deaths per year and 76,000 hospitalizations (9, 10).

The problem with medicine is two-fold. First, our society believes in medicine. Second, the industry makes billions of dollars and is under pressure to continue to do so.

Dr. Jay Cohen is one of the world's best authorities on the prescription drug business and author of "Over Dose: The Case Against the Drug Companies: Prescription Drugs, Side Effects, and Your Health," states that prescription drugs contribute to 300 U.S. deaths each day. One prominent reason is that the entire research and approval process for new drugs is less than a legitimate, upstanding process.

Dr. Cohen covers every in and out of the prescription drug business you would ever want to know. He states:

After more than a decade of research conducted without any influences, I found that the drug companies dominate the entire process of medication therapy – from early research to ultimate usage – as few other industries control their products today. Drug company research and development often serves marketing strategies more than sound science or patients' safety.

Dr. Cohen points out the following examples:

- Drug companies can conduct multiple studies on new drugs, and then select and publish the most favorable ones while suppressing the rest.
- Drug companies underwrite 70 percent of all medication research today. This gives the pharmaceutical industry tremendous power over the entire medication research effort, including the threat of lawsuits or loss of future funding for physicians wanting to publish unfavorable findings.
- The drug companies' influence even extends to the FDA... Experts with drug company ties fill many important advisory positions at the FDA. An investigation by USA Today found that more than half of the experts on FDA advisory committees "have financial relationships with the pharmaceutical companies that will be helped or hurt by their decisions."

Meanwhile, who knows how many deaths they indirectly contribute to by veering people toward an over-dependency on their quick fixes and away from a preventative and curative approach to health?

A big company has one job and one job only: to make money. I would say that drug companies have mastered it when they average 15 to 20 percent profit margins annually. Did you know that the largest companies in the world like oil companies and food store chains only average about a 3 percent profit margin? Drug companies often make over five times that profit percentage. Recently, the top 10 drug companies in the United States had a median profit margin of 17 percent, compared with only 3.1 percent for all the other industries on the Fortune 500 list (11).

The fundamental belief within the medical system is that when the human body malfunctions you can fix the body by treating the malfunction. I have to say this is reasonable logic if you think of the human body as a machine in which the whole is equal to the sum of its parts.

Let's break this down, if you have an organ that malfunctions or goes bad, then replace it or repair it and you may just fix the problem. If you have tests that measure chemicals in the body, and you know what the normal range for those chemicals should be, then you could use drugs to get those chemicals within normal ranges. Makes sense, right? Wrong, remember the human body performs over 360 trillion chemical reactions every minute. Each is one perfectly timed to be in harmony and collaboration with every other chemical reaction. This balance is dangerously upset by outside, manmade, toxic and powerful drugs. This is the reason every drug ever created has multiple side effects.

In addition, you have doctors who genuinely want to help people. And if the only tools the doctor has are what he was taught, which is drugs or surgery, what recommendation do you think the person is going to get? The doctor believes they have succeeded because they helped a person not have pain.

Of course things get much more complicated because the doctor is not helping the person by treating the pain or the symptoms. Doing that ignores the origin or cause of the problem.

Let's look at two human bodies that have all their original parts intact. One of these bodies is alive and the other one is dead. Both of these bodies have all of their internal organs, no fluids are missing from either of the bodies, both bodies have a brain and heart, etc. No matter how alike both of these bodies are physically there is something very different about these bodies, and that something cannot be weighed or physically removed. A human body that has all of its parts and a body that is animated by a vital living force, is very different from a body that has all of its parts but is not living. A human body that is equal to the sum of its parts is represented by the dead body; it has all of its parts and yet it is dead. The human body that has all of its parts and is alive is greater than just the sum of its parts. This is the difference when thinking vitalistically.

When you understand that the nervous system controls every function of the body, and that disturbance to nerve communication has a negative effect on body function, you quickly realize that the central nervous system plays a critical role in the daily health and function of your body. Wouldn't it then seem logical to look to the nervous system as a starting point for all malfunctions in someone's health? Of course it would make sense to at least start there even if you don't end up finding the problem in the nervous system. Instead you hear stories about doctors treating people's symptoms and people never getting well because they constantly take drugs to cover up the side effects of those symptoms. And then they take more drugs to cover up the side effects of those symptoms. Taking drugs rarely, if ever, can lead to more wellness long term. The chemical strain on the body is just too much. Drugs are powerful chemicals that are best used as short term solutions to getting your health on the right track so that you no longer need the drug. I would define short term as less than two years.

The dangers of medical drugs are not lost on many doctors. It has been reported that up 75 percent of doctors would refuse chemotherapy for cancer treatment (12). ABC news reports that only 60 percent of doctors and nurses would receive a flu shot (13). I personally know pediatricians, who asked to be made anonymous, who have said that they refused to vaccinate their children with any childhood vaccines. These doctors say that the risks of the vaccines are just too great to outweigh any possible short-term benefits. They argue that childhood vaccines have only limited short term effects and never provide life long immunity against diseases.

What I want you to do to begin to Live SuperHuman is to start thinking about your body differently than you've ever thought about before. I want you to think about your body as living, vital, amazing and powerful at all times. I want you to know that the power that made your body is the same power that heals your body and if you can maximize that power, it is one of the easiest ways to stay strong and healthy.

Chapter 22

Heart Attacks And Cholesterol

Because it's the third leading cause of death in the country, I'd like to spend more time talking about heart disease and how you can change your lifestyle to prevent it.

A heart attack occurs when the small blood vessels that supply the actual heart muscle with oxygen become clogged. When that happens, blood no longer nourishes the muscle that beats your heart and it dies. When the muscle dies it traumatizes the rhythm and coordination of the heartbeat, which can stop the heart completely and kill you. Not SuperHuman!

How do the small blood vessels get clogged? Here is where the disagreements in healthcare start. Many medical doctors believe the source of a heart attack is that cholesterol clogs up blood vessels and that blockage gives people heart attacks. Doctors believe this because they can cut open a blood vessel and test the material clogging it and see that it is cholesterol. It seems pretty straight forward right? If you stop right here and don't use your SuperHuman brain, that is what you might believe. The real question is, why is cholesterol clogging up this blood vessel?

Cholesterol is a very, very important part of not only our bodies but the entire world. Simply, cholesterol is made of two parts: fat and protein. That's it—not good and bad cholesterol as some people might say. Fat and protein are joined together in the liver to make cholesterol, which is used as a transport vehicle in your watery blood. What makes this chemical so important is that in order to survive, you must have lots of it. Pounds and pounds of cholesterol make up much of our bodies. Every cell has an outer layer called a cell wall. Every cell in your body, over 100 trillion of them, have walls derived from cholesterol. Nearly every cell wall of every living creature on earth is made of cholesterol.

Many of the chemicals that regulate your body are made from cholesterol, like hormones. All hormones are made from cholesterol components and perform critical actions like regulating wake and sleep cycles, determining reproductive cycles, affecting your mood, regulating your energy levels, and so on. Cholesterol also plays a vital role in facilitating healing processes and tissue repair. Now that you understand how important cholesterol is the next logical question is, "How is it considered so bad?" I'll answer that for you now.

Since cholesterol is made up of just fat and protein and nothing more it can't be good or bad. What you have to know is what the environment is like inside your blood vessels. Imagine for a minute that you and I are going to go on a tour of the inside of your blood vessels. We magically shrink down to the size of a cell, which is hundreds of times smaller than the period at the end of this sentence, and we are transported into your own blood stream. In here it is a crazy and fast-paced place like Times Square in New York City squished down with a 10-foot ceiling on top. Everything happens at an unbelievable pace and we are caught in the forceful current of your blood rushing us down and through your vessels like pinballs at the mercy of the forceful pressure. We are bounced to and fro, crashing into other cells and banging into the walls of the vessel itself. We are pushed hurriedly forward by the rushing current for a moment and then the powerful rush of watery blood slows slightly before we are helplessly pushed forward again with no control over what we collide with.

Hopefully this gives you a little bit of an image of what it is like in your blood stream. It is a violent, high-pressure system that is completely sealed and necessary to keep you alive. That is why there is a measurement of your blood pressure. This chaotic system is what makes cholesterol potentially damaging. Remember there is no such thing as good or bad cholesterol, there is just fat and protein. What makes it potentially damaging is the size and density of the molecule itself. High density lipoproteins, or HDL's, called "good" cholesterol by medicine, and low density lipoproteins, or LDL's, called "bad" cholesterol by medicine. Other than drug company marketing, this is where the perception of good and bad comes from. One theory is that if the molecule is small and dense, like a hard little pinball, it can be driven right into the walls of the blood vessel by the force of the pressure and tear it open. If the molecule is larger, it is less likely to cause any damage to the muscular wall of the vessel. When a hard little cholesterol molecule tears open the vessel wall, an entire healing process is started.

Remember, cholesterol is used to aid in the healing process. Therefore, whenever you have damage or inflammation in an area of the body, cholesterol is shuttled to that area right away. If you have inflammation throughout your body due to an illness, obesity, general poor health or chronic pain (which all increase systemic inflammation) then you will have extra cholesterol running through your vessels. This will increase the chances that you will have more of the small, dense pinballs tearing up your vessel walls.

These little tears happen all the time and your body is prepared for it in a major way. You have an entire system specifically designed to heal up damage to blood vessel walls. First, cholesterol is rushed to the tear to patch it up by covering and clogging it up while other cells of the wall repair the tear—like a cut in your skin that develops a scab while the underlying damage is repaired. When the damage is finally repaired, special white blood cells go to the area and gobble up the cholesterol patch and transport the cholesterol back to the liver for reuse (another sign that cholesterol is important is that it is constantly recycled). This process of removing cholesterol from the blood vessel walls happens constantly in your body. The big problem occurs when free radicals oxidize the cholesterol before it can be transported back to the liver.

A basic chemistry review will help you understand free radicals and oxidation. The stability of an atom or molecule (more than one atom bonded together) depends upon the number of electrons in the outer orbit of the atom or molecule. When the electrons in the outer orbit are paired, or come in sets of two, the molecule is more stable and less likely to react with other atoms or molecules. Free radicals are atoms, molecules, or ions with a single unpaired electron on the outer orbit. These unpaired electrons are usually highly reactive, seeking to find another electron to pair with in order to stabilize the atom or molecule. These reactions are called "oxidizing" and a common example is what happens to bananas or apples that are left out in the air and turn brown. Therefore, free radicals are likely to take part in chemical reactions. Radicals play an important role in biochemistry and many chemical processes, including human chemical function.

Free radicals are suspected culprits in causing the aging process in humans like wrinkles, gray hair and the general decline in health that people can experience as they age. If you could prevent the build up of free radicals in your body, then you could potentially slow down your aging process dramatically. That would be a SuperHuman power we all want to have!

When the cholesterol in your blood encounters one of these highly reactive free radicals, it becomes oxidized, changing its normal chemical makeup. This change turns your normal, helpful cholesterol into a sticky, goopy substance that inflames the lining of your blood vessels and traps the white blood cells trying to remove it. Imagine it changing from a clay-like texture to rubber cement. This inflammation only adds to the problem and begins to clog the vessel even faster. Ultimately this is what causes a heart attack. According to author and metabolic medicine expert Dr. Ron Rosedale, too much cholesterol is not the cause of a heart attack. The connection between heart disease and cholesterol exists mostly because of the volume of cholesterol flowing through your arteries and veins due to your current state of health. Otherwise there would be little or no connection between heart disease and cholesterol.

If you could prevent cholesterol from becoming sticky, goopy, oxidized, rubber cement clinging to your arterial walls and allow your white blood cells to do their job and remove cholesterol build up, then you would have a more powerful way of preventing heart attacks and heart disease.

This is the new superpower that I want to give you: a way that you can be more powerful in preventing heart disease in yourself

and your family members and loved ones. Knowing the connection between heart disease and cholesterol gives you a power that you otherwise did not have. It also gives you a huge clue as to which nutritional supplements will benefit you the most in preventing heart disease and heart attacks.

Live SuperHuman Tool: **A major cause of heart attacks is the fact that when cholesterol is oxidized it builds up in your arteries faster. Prevent heart attacks with nutritional supplements designed to prevent oxidation. Reduce total cholesterol levels in your blood by following other SuperHuman lifestyle tips recommended in this book.**

Did you know that the best selling drugs of all time are drugs claiming to lower cholesterol (14)? Lipitor is the highest selling drug in the history of medicine. Lipitor does more than $9 billion in sales per year. (That's more than $1 million per hour every hour of every day 365 days per year)! Lipitor is in a class of drugs called statins. Statin drugs work by inhibiting an enzyme vital in the formation process of cholesterol. Blocking this enzyme creates potential for numerous side effects because the production of cholesterol requires a sequence of many steps. Each step is a chemical reaction that produces byproducts used by the body in other processes. A huge problem is created by statin drugs because this vital process is stopped in the first few steps.

Lipitor's warning insert lists nearly 130 side effects I have listed 34 of them for you. **I want you to read this list carefully** and think about how many other problems could be caused in one's life by these side effects: chest pain, fever, neck rigidity, malaise, nausea, vomiting, rectal hemorrhage, mouth ulceration, anorexia, stomach ulcer, hepatitis, pneumonia, insomnia, dizziness, uncoordination, peripheral neuropathy, facial paralysis, depression, arthritis, leg cramps, dry skin, acne, eczema, urinary tract infection, urinary frequency, eye hemorrhage, deafness, glaucoma, taste loss, migraine, hypertension, weight gain, hypoglycemia and rhabdomyolysis, also known as muscle breakdown.

You would think that any one of these side effects would be enough to scare someone away from taking these drugs. Think of all the other medication that might be prescribed to handle the symptom of the side effect. Think of all the car accidents that could be caused by people who are slightly tired, dizzy, depressed, having vision and muscle control coordination problems? This stuff affects people's lives dramatically.

Even scarier is that you don't know which one of these problems you are most likely to get until the damage is already done and you have started experiencing the dis-ease or symptoms. I know what you are thinking; "I understand Dr. Rook, and I know these drugs are bad for me, but isn't that better than dying from a heart attack?" What you are saying to me is that the only reason you would take one of these drugs is to prevent a heart attack. Your answer has already been researched by many scientists and I'm happy to share the information they have found with you.

Research studies like the December 2002 issue of the Journal of the American Medical Association show that these drugs may lower your blood cholesterol levels but they have **no effect** on whether or not you have a heart attack. Studies show that taking these drugs gives you absolutely ZERO protection from having a heart attack. This research further validates that cholesterol levels are not the major factor in determining if you will have a heart attack or not.

Now this is where I get extremely passionate about the cholesterol and heart disease issue. Earlier we talked about what hormones are made of: cholesterol which is a primary source for hormone building blocks. Well what do you think happens to your ability to make hormones when all these drugs enter someone's body and artificially block cholesterol production? Your hormone production goes down as well.

Serotonin is a hormone that helps determine things like appetite, sleep and mood or how happy you are. You could call it a feel-good hormone. Healthy levels of serotonin will allow a person to have a more stable mood, be happier, avoid depression and have a more positive outlook style. All things that you want to have in abundance when living a SuperHuman life. When someone's serotonin levels get too low it can cause or contribute to many horrible problems. Research studies show that low levels of mood stabilizing hormones are associated with problems like depression, violence, arson, suicide and even homicide (15). The world becomes a more dangerous, violent and unhappy place when our bodies cannot function the way they are naturally intended to.

It breaks my heart to think that there are kids who aren't as close to their dads, and wives that don't feel loved, men who can't figure out why they can't be who they used to be, and families broken apart by something that can be so simply prevented by living as I have outlined for you. Please share what you know because you are now more educated on these issues than most everyone you know. Don't keep any information you have read a secret. I feel that we are morally obligated to make the world better for those around us. Naturally it will make our own world much better.

A very strong example of how you could become a direct victim of one of these drug effects—even if you're not on them yourself—was brought to light by the American Heart Association. At a 2005 meeting of the association attendees discussed findings that people who are taking statin drugs have substantially slower nerve reaction times. Imagine that someone taking one of these drugs is driving but cannot react in time to stop their car and they crash into you or your kids. I don't even want to think how often some type of accident like this happens. An accident that may have been prevented by something as small as healthy cholesterol levels unaltered by a drug.

Live SuperHuman Tool: **SuperHumans know they have the power to help save others. They never doubt this power and act decisively to share it with others. I believe that I can help you learn how to do exactly that. Share the information with others, so that you, too, can help save others.**

This is a perfect explanation of why I had to write this book: to give us all a way to help each other in making the world a much better, safer, happier and healthier place. A place where all people are super heroes looking out for one another. By living healthier and sharing this information with as many people as we can, together, we can literally have a life-saving, positive impact on our communities that spreads quickly and powerfully.

Chapter 23

Bad Supplements Can Kill You

Live SuperHuman Tool: **Fighting diseases is a superpower! Take multiple kinds of top quality antioxidants and the best multi vitamins to strengthen your disease fighting super powers.**

For heart health it is important that we address omega fatty acids. Fish Oil has become one of the most popular supplements on the planet and for good reason! Of all the nutritional supplements you can take, fish oil is the only one I've ever seen that continues to receive more and more supportive good press and evidence to take it. Granted, you want to get it from quality sources that eliminate your intake of toxins. Fish that live long lives and grow to larger sizes will accumulate more poisonous toxins, like mercury, than will smaller, short-life fish. Be aware that not all fish oils are created equally and if your fish oil is made with inexpensive ingredients, it may mean that you are paying the price with toxins.

Two key nutrients in fish oil help give you disease fighting superpowers: EPA and DHA. Eicosapentanoic Acid (EPA) is found in fish, which get it from micro algae they feed on. It is also found in spirulina, a type of algae known as a superfood due to its powerful nutritional content, and breast milk. EPA has been shown to deliver incredible anti-inflammatory power to your body, helping to keep your blood from clogging your heart arteries. It has also been shown to help schizophrenia, depression, and prevent certain types of cancers (16, 17, 18, 19, 20, 21).

The other special nutrient in fish oil is DHA or docosahexanoic acid. DHA is particularly important to the health and development of the brain and nervous system. It is the most abundant fatty acid found in the brain and retina of the eye, making it important for vision as well. DHA is being studied in human trials to see how well it battles Alzheimer's disease. It also has been shown to help fight depression, colon and prostate cancer (22, 23, 24, 25, 26, 27).

The next supplement you absolutely must take in order to Live SuperHuman are antioxidants. Antioxidants are one of the most powerful and life saving nutrients you can possibly take to help prevent the aging process, the oxidizing of cholesterol and the clogging of your blood vessels. They can help prevent heart attacks better than any drug ever could. I'm going to give you a very specific list of antioxidants I take every day that I believe you should take also. I take three primary categories of antioxidants: 1. whole-food greens, fruits and superfoods, 2. oligomeric proanthocyanidins found in fruits, berries and pine bark and 3. exotic fruit xanthones. There is literally a mountain of science that explains the incredible whole-body benefits of these three groups of antioxidants. In my mind, there is no doubt that these create the strongest antioxidant combination to fight against aging and deadly diseases.

I searched dozens of companies and literally thousands of products over a decade to try to find a cost effective and efficient way to deliver all these nutrients to my patients. What I found was the same disappointment everywhere. I had to go to many different companies to find the products people needed and all of them were very expensive. That translated into a person having to buy many different products at a hefty cost. I was not happy with that because it is inefficient and expensive—not the SuperHuman way.

After years of trying different combinations of nutritional supplements, I've found a number of products that work very well. Unfortunately, I always had to get them from different sources. Over time that process became very frustrating, especially knowing that a client was paying literally five to 10 times the price of what they could be paying if all these nutritional supplements were combined into one formula. It was this frustration that inspired me to create a unique nutritional supplement that combined all of the powerful nutrients and formulas people need to help them Live SuperHuman.

Many nutritional supplement companies will not sell you a supplement unless you are a licensed healthcare provider. I had to create a nutritional supplement from a combination of supplements I have access to as a doctor. I started mixing these supplements together and calling it my "SuperHuman Drink." Part of my morning routine is always mixing these supplements together in a glass, adding water and stirring it all up so that I could start the day with my SuperHuman supplement. My son and daughter both began drinking this formula when they were well under 8 years old. To this day my son asks me every morning, "Dad, can I have a SuperHuman Drink?" This should tell you that not only is this drink exceptionally yummy, but teaching kids healthy habits is one way to ensure they will Live SuperHuman as they develop and be "strong and healthy" as we like to say in my family.

The best part is that now my kids wake up every morning and tell me they want their SuperHuman Drink. If they don't get their drink, trust me, they let me know. It has become part of our morning routine and, proudly, I have begun to teach them how they can be SuperHuman from an early age. This is so easy to do that any family could implement this strategy into their family health routine right now and have it catch on.

We all know that spending money on your health is a worthy investment. However, you still have to be able to afford to buy other things you need to be as healthy as you want to be. I like to tell my patients that you can't choose between buying groceries to feed your family and buying nutritional supplements or getting chiropractic care. However, when it's not in your budget to spend $175 on antioxidants, but it is in your budget to spend a fraction of that, it makes a big difference. Remember, you are investing now with the intent to avoid having to deal with future health conditions and related costs.

I have found that a complete line of nutritional supplements a family needs is hard to get within a comfortable price range. What I have people do is bring me a list of their supplements, and I'll do an audit on that list. I'm amazed at the number of supplements people take—sometimes 10, 20 or 30 individual products every day. Not only is it inconvenient, but that is a lot of pills! I usually find that people are duplicating many of their nutrients and can eliminate some.

Recently, I consulted with a woman who was spending about $100 per month on just her multivitamin product. To me that was just preposterous. Right now, I am going to teach you ways to get all of your supplements by taking very few pills, spending very little money, and getting all the nutrients you need to create your SuperHuman body and health.

Now that you know all about the causes of cancer and heart disease, you are an expert on cholesterol, and you want to avoid doctor visits and drugs whenever possible by boosting your immune system to super strength, I'm going to share with you the three basic supplements you must take.

1. You must have a multivitamin that contains whole-food-sourced, fermented nutrients. Whole-food-sourced fermented nutrients are closer to their natural state and pre-metabolized in the fermentation process. This allows them to be assimilation-ready and therefore absorbed up to 200 times more easily than old fashioned isolated nutrient supplements. A multivitamin is critical because nutrients always work more effectively when they can synergize with other nutrients. It is rarely more beneficial for your body to take individual vitamins and minerals.

2. You must take in enough antioxidants to fight off all of the inflammation, cancer causing and cholesterol oxidizing damage that happens to you on a daily basis. The very best antioxidants come in the form of super foods such as whole food greens, fruits and vegetables, exotic fruits, and resveratrol. The supplement should contain nutrients that protect your skin to help you look younger, boost your energy and vitality, boost your immune

system to protect you from disease, as well as deliver all this to you at once or you'll have to waste money on separate products.

3. The final supplement you should take is fish oil or krill oil product. The critical nutrients in fish and krill oil are called EPA and DHA.

I believe that with the right recommendations you should be able to get all of these supplements at a very affordable price. At first, to build up your SuperHuman power you may need to take a higher dose of all of these supplements, but after a few weeks or months as your body gets stronger you would be able to reduce the amount of the supplements that you take in. And it makes sense if you think about it—as your level of wellness increases the amount of work it takes to stay there will decrease. It is just like I tell my patients: "As you get better, you should need fewer of my services until you find a happy level of wellness care that works for you."

Chapter 24

Never Sick...No Problem

One of the primary goals of this book is to teach you ways you can take charge of your own health. Super health makes it much easier to take care of other people and help them become SuperHuman, too. You are learning ways that you can be independent and free from having to rely on others to tell you how to live your life.

On the topic of nutrients I want to share with you a powerful secret that many doctors use to help people fight off sicknesses. When your immune system is depressed, viruses and other agents that under normal circumstances wouldn't make you sick can take hold and cause illnesses. Those illnesses can range from mild, like the common cold, to more severe, like the flu or worse. Having a strong immune system is the only way to ensure you can fight off illness. The secret I'm about to share with you, this tool, is based on the work of one of the most influential chemists in history, someone who ranks among the most important scientists in any field of the 20th century.

Dr. Linus Pauling, who died in 1994 at the age of 93, outlived the life expectancy of people of his generation by nearly 50 years through education and healthy habits. Dr. Pauling is the only person to have been awarded multiple Nobel Prizes without sharing it with another recipient. His work is the foundation for this immune building secret and something I am excited to share with you here.

Dr. Pauling conducted extensive studies on the efficacy of Vitamin C, taken in large doses, to ward off the common cold. His conclusion proved that not only did large amounts of Vitimin C prevent illness, but that previous findings, which concluded that the body simply could not process more than 100 grams of the vitamin a day, was erroneous. Overall, Dr. Pauling suggested that Vitamin C is a vital component of good health and at the first sign of sickness, people should increase their intake.

It's amazingly simple, according to Dr. Pauling. I want you to understand these important points before I tell you what you could do for yourself because I want you to understand there is Nobel Prize winning authority behind it. The first point is that vitamin C has a powerful effect on the immune system. The second, is that taking a lot of vitamin C is not harmful or wasteful. Third, it's important to know that vitamin C can improve the strength of your immune system so much so that it can prevent you from getting sick.

Almost everyone has a noticeable change in their body when they start to get run down from sickness. It's the subtle change that occurs before you actually get the first signs of being sick. For some people it is becoming very tired. For others it is being increasingly emotional. For me and other people I know, my body alerts me to impending illness with a sore throat.

The only time I have been sick in the last decade occurred a few years ago. I was divorced, my business was building, and I was in between staff to help me in my office, so I was in the process of hiring and training someone. I had recently met my future wife and was falling in love so I was staying up late and getting up early nearly every day for weeks. After a while my body gave me the warning sign that I was pushing too hard in the form of a sore throat. I know that warning sign very well so I listened. I was still working hard, however, I made sure to get to bed earlier, take my vitamins, and rest more on my off days. Within a couple of days my sore throat was gone and I felt great. So, what did I do? I went right back at it of course. Pushing, getting little sleep and thinking I'd get away with it. Not more than a few days later a sore throat came on again and so did the rest of the signs and symptoms of a viral infection. I only came down with what some people would call a bad cold or a slight flu that lasted 48 hours, however, that was the first time I had been sick in about seven years.

If you can't say that you have only been sick one time in the last 10 years then my suggestion to you is follow every piece of advice that's written in this book starting today and in the next 10 to 15 years you will be able to say that.

Here is what I do and have recommended to many patients successfully: at the first signs of being run down—not being sick just run down—start taking vitamin C three times per day, 3,000 to 5,000 mg each time. So you could take a total of around 15,000 mg of vitamin C per day, whether you actually get sick or not, until you feel better. Do not take vitamin C on a regular basis except for what is already included in your daily SuperHuman supplements. It is very difficult to overdose on vitamin C and the first sign that people get, like Dr. Pauling says, is a laxative effect. If this happens then reduce the amount of vitamin C take until you no longer experience it. I have seen this little piece of advice, combined with chiropractic adjustments, work literally hundreds of times in either preventing a sickness completely or reducing the length and severity of the sickness by about 50 percent.

Chapter 25

Injecting Poison

One of the most controversial issues in healthcare right now is that of vaccinations, particularly childhood vaccinations and flu shots. Flu shots are disturbing to me. Every year you hear the fear mongering in the news, recommending that everybody needs to get a flu shot, including children and pregnant women. Also, everyone needs to do it in a hurry because the flu is coming and it might get you—or they might run out of vaccines before you get your chance. We turn elementary schools into vaccination clinics. Every year you hear the stories about people who are at risk or going to die from a new strain of the flu like the Bird Flu, Swine or some other seasonal flu.

Can you imagine the uproar that would occur if schools were turned into chiropractic clinics and kids were supposed to get a proven safe adjustment on a specific day or else be at risk from a health problem? Yet people allow chemicals to be injected into their kids at school with little argument. This is appalling to me.

What you don't hear much fuss about is how in recent years (2004, 2007, 2008), the CDC admits that they missed the mark while creating the flu vaccine and didn't put the right flu virus strain components in the vaccine (28). The CDC reports that "the majority (66 percent) of influenza A (H1N1) viruses were found to be similar to the vaccine strain. However, **77 percent** of influenza A (H3N2) and **98 percent** of B viruses sent to CDC for further testing were not optimally matched to the 2007-08 influenza vaccine strains." (29)

Interpretation: the flu shot did not help you up to 98 percent of the time.

This means that millions of people were vaccinated with a flu shot that didn't even contain the ingredients necessary to fight the flu virus that was circulating.

If we look at it closely and really think about what's going on, we realize quickly that the aftermath of something like the Bird Flu or even the Swine Flu is extremely minimal. The book "The Great Bird Flu Hoax" by Dr. Joe Mercola became a New York Times Bestseller because people want the truth. As a matter of fact when it comes right down to it, all of that hype seems to be blowing something out of proportion that we never should have worried about the first place.

In June 2009 my wife and I, in the height of the Swine Flu scare, went to Mexico for a vacation just south of Cancun. What we saw was not a lively Mexican culture known for celebration and hospitality but a culture that had been devastated by a decline in tourism. This area of the Yucatán Peninsula is one of the most beautiful places in the world. It attracts millions of tourists year-round. The local people rely on the tourism economy to sustain their jobs and their lives. When talking with one of the employees at the resort we stayed at, we were told that the resort was actually 50 percent shutdown at the time and they had laid off some 600 workers due to the downturn in travelers run off by the Swine Flu scare. There may have been other factors involved but the perception of local people was that swine flu was to blame.

That is 600 people without jobs from only one resort! Just think how many people lost their jobs and are now struggling to help their families. This is heartbreaking to me. I was also infuriated that the mass media would scare people to the point that it would devastate an economy so that drug companies can make more money.

At that time, as of June 12, 2009, 74 countries had officially reported 29,669 cases of influenza A(H1N1) infection and only 145 deaths in the entire world from this illness. The United States had 13,217 confirmed cases and 27 deaths. Mexico has had fewer cases but still had the majority of the deaths at 108. That gave someone roughly a

.000059 percent chance of catching the flu and a .49 percent chance of dying if they did get sick.

A 2010 review of the Cochrane Database for influenza vaccine results, including 50 reports, forty of them clinical trials with over 70,000 people, came to the conclusion there is **no value in any influenza vaccine!** It states over 200 viruses cause influenza or flu like symptoms, so at best the flu vaccine may affect 10 percent of all these viruses. Vaccine use did not affect hospitalization or work days lost. Live aerosol vaccines, whether or not they guessed right on which virus the vaccine contains, had minimal effectiveness, less than 10 percent. There is NO EVIDENCE vaccines affect complications from the flu or transmission of the virus! The results of this review discourage the use of vaccination against the flu (30). And I couldn't have said it better myself!

At LiveSuperHuman.com you can find many more vaccination resources and download an ebook called The Swine Flu Hoax: 50 Billion Reasons Not to Get a Flu Shot! The is the reason I wrote this book is so you could see, in detail, answers to questions about the insanity of the flu shot industry. This book will for sure help you make up your mind on what is the right thing for you to do.

This is a question that I get asked all the time: "Dr. Rook, should I get a flu shot?" When I answer this question, I actually don't share my opinion. The way I answer this question is by quoting an immunologist explaining the way that the immune system reacts to the flu shot when you are vaccinated. This is how it was explained to me and I absolutely loved this explanation because it made total sense to me.

Live SuperHuman Tool: **Do everything you can to avoid getting a flu shot.**

You may know someone who has received a flu shot and a few days later got sick from the flu. Then you hear that person say, "I am never getting a flu shot again." This is how it was explained to me that can happen:

First, you must understand that the flu shot is one of the only vaccines that still carries or can carry a live virus. Some shots have weakened virus or killed virus, but you may or may not even know what you're getting. When you get vaccinated with a flu shot, that flu shot contains a particular virus. Let's call it virus A. That virus begins to take hold in your body by entering a cell and multiplying. The cell that is infected alerts your immune system that it contains a virus of a specific nature. Your immune system proceeds to build up cells designed to fight that particular virus type. Your immune cells then surround the infected cell and wait for the virus to multiply so much that it kills the cell and ruptures it. When these viruses, thousands of them, burst out of the cell your waiting immune system cells begin to gobble up the fleeing viruses. However, a few lucky viruses sneak away and infect other cells. Then the whole process starts over.

Eventually these viruses, which have their own living, adapting, innate intelligence, realize they are losing this battle. Since viruses can multiply so quickly, they can go through generations and make genetic changes in a very short period of time. Their programming for survival leads them to change their genetic code so they are now virus B instead of virus A. Your immune system has been programmed only with cells that fight virus A and therefore, is unable to recognize or fight virus B very effectively. Virus B now affects your body and the resulting infection is what makes you sick.

This is how someone gets sick from the flu shot. They actually get sick with a different flu than the one they were vaccinated for. Another possible way people get sick from a flu shot is that the chemicals in the shot weaken a person's immune system enough to allow them to get sick, rather than stay strong enough to fight off the virus.

Chapter 26

Childhood Vaccinations: Blind Shots

Now that we've talked about flu vaccinations, let's talk about childhood vaccinations, which are another issue altogether. Many books have touched on this topic and to read them all, you'd need literally hundreds of hours to educate yourself. By educated, I mean that you have fully taken the time to become aware of the theory behind why vaccinations are recommended and you are 100 percent knowledgeable on all of the possible negative effects of the childhood vaccine.

The arguments to vaccinate are well known, unchanged, outdated and do not need further discussion. For the purposes of this book I will only illustrate my favorite reasons against vaccination, which are the ones based on logic and are the easiest to understand. They are also, I believe, the best starting point in your education. These points include:

1. Children are not supposed to receive childhood vaccinations if they have a weakened or compromised immune system or have a genetic predisposition that might cause them to react badly to a vaccine. This makes total sense, however, children rarely receive proper testing to diagnose immune system or genetic deficiencies before they are given shots.

2. The ingredients in vaccines are a concoction of poison that no one in their right mind—not even any drug company executive—

would be willing to inject into their own body adjusted for weight. Jock Doubleday, director of Natural Woman, Natural Man, Inc., currently offers $250,000 to the first medical doctor, pharmaceutical company CEO, or ACIP member who publicly drinks a mixture of standard vaccine additive ingredients in the same dosage a 6-year-old child is recommended to receive under the year-2005 guidelines of the U.S. Centers for Disease Control and Prevention. (31). These ingredients include African green monkey kidney cells, alcohol, aluminum oxide, ammonium sulfate, aspartame, chick embryo cells, Chinese hamster ovary cells, ethylene glycol, ethylenediaminetetraacetic (EDTA), formaldehyde, human diploid cells (aborted fetal disuse), monosodium glutamate, neomycin, phenol, squalene, sucrose, mercury, and about 200 other toxic ingredients.

3. The number of vaccine doses recommended for children in the first few years of life now totals more than 49! There is no scientific justification, research or proof that pouring this many chemicals into a child's body and underdeveloped immune system is safe.

4. Childhood vaccinations are experimental. Do you really think it's ethical to test the effects of these powerful drugs and ingredients on unsuspecting children and babies?

5. Why is there a secretive court that hears cases for vaccine injured children that keeps all records sealed permanently? All vaccine claims are managed and adjudicated by the congressionally-created Office of Special Masters and provides drug companies with a questionable three-year statute of limitations provision severely limiting children's rights to compensation for long term damage. It can be argued that these children are not offered equal constitutional protection as other injured parties.

6. Why have vaccine makers been indemnified from having to pay unlimited monetary damages to those injured by their products when other companies have full liability and an open end to the possible damages they may have to pay out?

7. Death rates from all diseases such as polio, measles, mumps, rubella, pertussis, and diphtheria declined by over 95 percent between 1850 and 1946, long before mass vaccination was implemented in the 1950's. This decline occurred because of and in conjunction with improved sanitation and hygiene standards in industrialized nations.

8. I know these diseases all sound terrible but the fact is that they are all classified as "self-limiting diseases," which means that most of the time people get sick for a period and then get well on their own. The resulting effect is life long immunity. More susceptible people had severe effects from the diseases or died, like the flu, from which most people get sick and then get well. Very few people in higher risk categories die every year from these conditions in proportion. SuperHumans rarely, if ever, get sick or die from conditions like these.

9. In nature, diseases don't get injected directly into your blood stream, therefore, your immune system is not prepared for that. What really happens is your mucous membranes (like in your sinuses) identify the intruder first, which sets off a cascade of events that creates life-long immunity. Bypassing this system creates a weak temporary immune reaction.

10. Vaccines don't provide life long immunity. The typical maximum immune reaction lasts about 5 years. "Boosters" don't actually boost the vaccine, they are a re-do for vaccine failure.

11. My new favorite: When in nature would anyone encounter or "catch" Hepatitis B, Polio, Measles, Mumps, Rubella, Diptheria, Pertussis, Tetanus, Chicken Pox, Cholera, Flu, Rotavirus, Meningitis, and Tuberculosis all at the same time (or even within one year)? Think about how ridiculous it is for a child's immune system to respond to that kind of an assault. You have better odds of winning a jackpot in the lottery than this happening to you. Literally you would have to step on a rusty nail covered in polio infested feces, get bit by a rabid dog, while injecting yourself with an infected IV drug needle, while sharing silverware at a meal with seven friends from undeveloped countries who have

> measles, mumps, diphtheria, rubella, cholera, meningitis and TB sealed in a room barely big enough to hold all of you without ventilation so you are required to breathe in each others' coughs and sneezes for 10 hours straight.

Why do they put all that stuff into a few vaccines and call it normal to inject it all right into your blood stream?

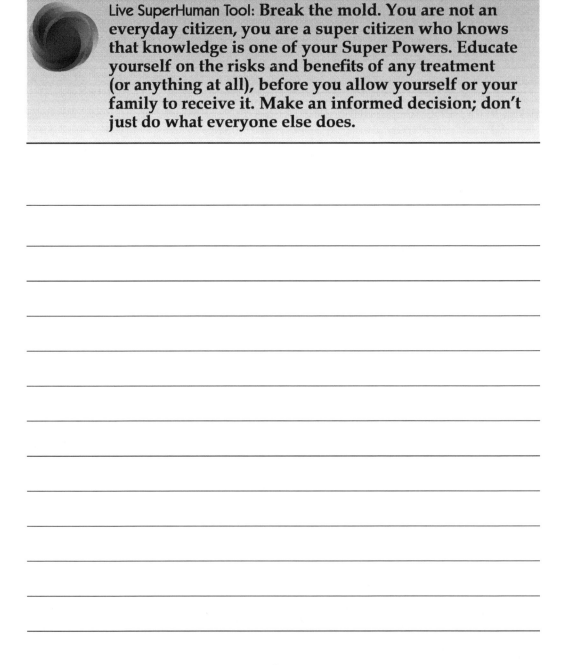

Live SuperHuman Tool: **Break the mold. You are not an everyday citizen, you are a super citizen who knows that knowledge is one of your Super Powers. Educate yourself on the risks and benefits of any treatment (or anything at all), before you allow yourself or your family to receive it. Make an informed decision; don't just do what everyone else does.**

Chapter 27

SuperHuman Elements of Wellness: Neuro-Spiritual

The term Neuro-Spiritual is a term that I developed specifically for this book to help you understand the concept that your nervous system is connected to your physical body and your spiritual self or mind-body connection. Dr. D.D. Palmer, known as the discoverer of chiropractic, used to say that the nervous system is what connects man the physical to man the spiritual. That was over 114 years ago and not only still rings true today but is being proven by scientific research. Talk about being ahead of your time!

In my chiropractic wellness center, and in the most advanced chiropractic clinics in the world, the doctors utilize technology called an Insight Subluxation Station. The reason for using an Insight is specifically to find subluxations. Subluxations are areas of the nervous system that have disturbance and are not working optimally or transmitting nerve signals optimally. Subluxations are what occur when stress accumulates from the nervous system continually trying to adapt the body to the massive amounts of stress that pound on us daily.

Considering that every cell, tissue and organ function of your body is controlled by the nervous system, that would mean that your health is 100 percent connected to the health of your nervous system. Being able to measure and optimize the health of your nervous system is the job of the chiropractor. Using the Insight I can measure the function of someone's nervous system so accurately that I can show you exactly where the nerve disturbance is and how bad it is.

The first test that I use is called a thermograph. If you are a patient in my office, the exact words I would tell you when you are going through the exam is this: "This test is called a thermograph, it measures temperature on both sides of your spine. Temperature is a direct reflection of blood flow at the skin surface and blood flow is controlled by the same part of your nervous system that controls your vital organs. This is called your autonomic nervous system, and this is a high-tech way to measure the nerve communication to your vital organs."

The next test I use is called a myograph and what I tell a patient during the exam is this: "This test is called a myograph. It measures the electrical voltage coming from your spinal cord out through your muscles. Therefore it measures the communication to your muscles. This part of your nervous system is called your motor nervous system."

The final test that I do is called a Pulse Wave Profile. This is my favorite test because it is so high-tech that all a person has to do is put their first three fingers inside a small sensor and within five minutes the sensor will determine how well their autonomic nervous system adapts their body to the environment. What I tell the patient is this: "This test is called a pulse wave profile and what it does is measure the communication between your brain and your heart, which have a special relationship. The communication between the brain and the heart is almost more intimate and constant than other parts of the body. What this test literally measures is the time between each heartbeat. The less that the time between each beat varies, the less adaptable you are and therefore less healthy you are. The more the time varies or changes between each beat, the healthier you are or the more adaptable you are. The more adaptable you are, the less susceptible you'll be to all diseases."

You probably didn't even know that this technology was available. However, knowing the health and the state of your nervous system is one of the most valuable tools that you can have when learning to Live SuperHuman.

Another technology I use for diagnosis and patient care in my office is a joint alignment and movement sensor. This technology is extremely advanced and utilizes a sensor that was developed by NASA for measuring the energetic vibration of the ceramic tiles on the bottom of the Space Shuttle. These tiles are used for cooling and dissipating heat as the Shuttle re-enters the earth's atmosphere at a speed greater than 28,000 km/h and about 1,500 degrees centigrade. This technology has been adapted for public use in areas like engineering and health care.

The sensor is so ultra sensitive that it can measure the vibrational movement and alignment of your spinal joints. Having healthy movement and alignment in the joints of your spine is critical to the health of your nervous system. When subluxations occur, one result may be that the joints of your spine can develop unhealthy movement or alignment. When this happens, the joints can start to decay, degenerate and age more quickly than they would if they had healthy movement and alignment. The best way to fix this problem is to have a chiropractic adjustment, which restores healthy movement and alignment allowing the nerve flow to return to optimal. This is different from a manipulation, which is designed to increase motion only and is performed by physical therapists or osteopaths.

The intent of a chiropractic adjustment is to have a positive impact on the nervous system, increase your GAP (Chapter 17), and therefore increase your human potential. You could say that chiropractors allow you to Live SuperHuman!

Now that you have learned so much about the 3 Elements of Wellness let's revisit the wellness scale. Imagine your health and wellness is measured on the scale below. The level zero represents sickness and death. The level above 150 represents your optimal wellness. The level 100 would be average. Each choice moves you down the scale toward zero or up the scale toward optimal wellness.

This is a very simple way to start taking steps to a healthier you right now. Every choice you make and action you take will move you in one direction or the other on the wellness scale. Right now, before reading on, circle where you think you are on the scale:

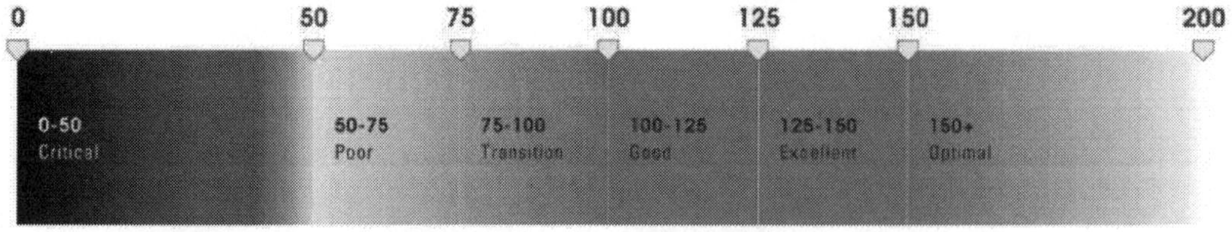

To move up the wellness scale, ask yourself if you've accomplished the following each day:

- Did I take my SuperHuman Drink today?
- Did I do my meditation this morning?
- Did I give the 5 Blessings to everyone I know and myself?
- Did I do Yoga today?
- Do I get my nerve system checked by a chiropractor consistently?
- Have I used a Super StretchTowel to strengthen my muscles today?
- Did what I eat today move me toward wellness?
- Have I replaced a bad habit with a good one?
- Did I eat a salad today?
- What goal did I set or reach today?

I know the greatest, most advanced wellness company in the world to be the Creating Wellness Alliance. They define wellness as "the degree to which an individual experiences health and vitality in any dimension of life." This definition states that wellness is not a destination but a constantly moving target. Wellness is a goal, if you will, that you constantly strive for and yet can never perfect. At any given moment in time, with every decision and choice you make, you are either moving toward wellness or away from it.

At Creating Wellness, they have actually created a name for your place on this scale. It is called your Wellness Quotient or WQ. There are a series of very advanced tests you can take to determine your actual WQ rather than guessing at it. These tests include checking to see if your nerve system is clear and healthy, determining how you process psychological stress, testing muscle strength, measuring vital lung capacity, calculating body composition and dozens more. This assessment is very affordable and every SuperHuman should have one performed annually at a minimum to keep track of their total wellness. At LiveSuperHuman.com we will help you keep track as well and even help you increase your WQ!

Section 4

Physical
Bio-chemical
Neuro-spiritual

Chapter 28

Purpose

One of the things that I know helps keep me extremely happy is that I live life with a purpose. That may sound cliché, and if you think so let me just ask you one question: What is your purpose? Have you ever thought about it or developed a purpose? You may even think it isn't important to have a purpose, but I can assure you it is not something you want to ignore.

This is why. Without defined purpose, how do you develop a value system through which to make every decision in your life? Your purpose molds the values that you use daily, and drives every action and decision you make. Without a defined purpose of your own, you end up with a purpose made up of a junk-pile of teachings, beliefs, thoughts, religions, rules, etc. from your environment. It's a disease in your body that has no specific origin, which comes from stress after stress that have piled up and left your body suffering and broken down.

You have this junk-pile purpose, whether you like it or not, think about it or not. No wonder so many people are confused, lost, struggling, unhealthy and unhappy, they have no internal purpose to drive their decision making. Developing a purpose from this mess can be very hard. And developing happiness from this mess can be even harder.

Trust me, I know how intimidating this can seem when you don't know where to start. It took me seven years to really define and refine my purpose. I can even tell you that if one of my greatest role models and mentors, Dr. Patrick Gentempo, had not led me to discover the importance of having a purpose, there is a very good chance that I would not have one to this day, and therefore not written this book for you. You see, this book, which took thousands of hours of training, thought, and work to produce, is a product of my purpose. My purpose is: **to lead my community to wellness.** How can I lead people to wellness if I'm not living wellness myself? I have a very disciplined routine for my wellness, much of which I'm teaching you here. So "my community" began with me personally. Then, "my community" became my family. Then "my community" became the city where I began my chiropractic wellness center, Boise, Idaho. I quickly realized that I was not thinking big enough and left out many people. I have relatives and friends in cities all over the country, all over the world! I couldn't leave them and their communities out, they are part of "my global community," and yet I can't be there in person leading them all to wellness all at the same time. However, through what I teach in this book and practice personally, I can expand my purpose, and create wellness in people across the globe. What an amazing gift that humbles and excites me, and you can do the same!

"I want a purpose," you say but how do you start? The very first thing I want you to know is this is quite easy. Look how short this next paragraph is. It may seem difficult because the concept of having or developing a purpose is so far out there to you. The simplest way for me to explain is to tell you what I did so you can let your own process unfold.

Ultimately your purpose statement should be short, simple and precise. The first question is: What do I want? Seriously, what do you want? Do you want happiness, love, health, wealth, or all of the above? Do you want these things you have selected for other people, too? Then make a statement such as, "I want to be happy and to make people happy." Simple and beautiful, that could be your purpose. When you decide on it, and you own it and it is truly who you are deep down, it becomes easy to live your life based on this purpose. When your commitment becomes who you are, every time you feel unhappy, you will move away from whatever is contributing to your unhappiness and move toward something which makes you happy.

The more you surround yourself with happiness, the more other people will notice and want to share in it with you. Do this and I guarantee you will be on your way to identifying what you want your purpose to be in life. Also know this: Once you determine, discover or create your purpose you will feel that it is right. It will resonate within you. You are likely to change over time and grow into a person who wants new things for yourself and the world, and when this happens, revisit your purpose and make sure the statement grows with you.

Chapter 29

Selflessness

The most amazing thing has happened to me and I can't really explain why. Perhaps it's because I had a lesson to learn. In any case, I want to address the issue of selflessness and selfishness. After observing a number of different situations, literally a dozens of them, I have come to notice that people seem to be extremely self-focused. I don't mean to say this in terms of being critical, I mean it simply as an observation. People's lives are so incredibly busy it forces them to focus on their own needs for the vast majority of the time. I don't think this is all bad, because I feel that it allows people to get the job done and meet the requirements they have to meet to get through each day. Things like pressures at work, getting kids from here to there, getting yourself from there to here, being on time, doing favors for others, getting yourself fed, taking care of yourself, getting the needs of your family met, your pets cared for, and getting yourself to bed, all put a heavy burden on an individual.

The main reason I want to bring this up is because I have noticed that someone else's self-focus can be a source of major stress for you personally if you are not careful. Remember that someone's attention or lack of attention to your needs is their business. Your attention to your needs is your business. Be careful not to point fingers or place blame on other people too quickly for not coming through for you or forgetting about your needs and wants. When you feel upset or angry or hurt because someone didn't come through for you or forgot about your needs it means you have taken it personally that you were not on the top of someone else's priority list. I realize that there are many times that we count on others to get the job done and help us out. But realize that everyone is often so focused on their own needs they may forget about yours, even if not intentionally. If this happens to you and you pout or get angry with them or feel any negative stress as a result of it, stop and think about who this hurts the most. Does all the negative energy that you feel inside, and the other person knows nothing about, hurt you the most or them? You of course.

I know there are literally hundreds to thousands of things to do everyday to meet your own needs, which makes it even more complicated and difficult. However, simply focusing a little attention on, and developing a sensitivity to, the needs of others will benefit you and them greatly. This is called compassion by some, and I have noticed lately that people just seem so focused on themselves that they forget the littlest things about the people around them who they love and care about. For example if your brother or sister told you about a small thing they really want as a gift, or as an experience, or just something that would help them out, would you be paying close enough attention during that conversation to remember in a week or a month what they had told you? What if they had told you that they were just under a lot of stress and you happened to be given a gift certificate for a massage or spa treatment, would you remember that there was someone in your life who could possibly benefit from that service more than you could? Or would you just go get it done for yourself without thinking of anyone else? Not that you should or shouldn't use it yourself, that isn't the point. The point is, ask yourself if you would think of others while you're thinking of yourself. If someone said they were pressed for time and they just needed some help, would you offer to get the oil changed in their car so they wouldn't have to run the extra errand?

I think it's so incredibly important that we as a society, as we learn to Live SuperHuman, learn to become more compassionate. By doing that, we develop a sensitivity for the needs of those around us. We should pay careful attention, not only our own needs, but the needs of those around us, so that we can do our best to remember them and meet them whenever we can. This may seem like a high expectation to a lot of people but hold on...

Think about if you had a number of friends and relatives who are doing this for you, would you have more time? Would you have less stress? Would you have less on your mind? Wouldn't this give you the ability to more easily pay attention to the needs of others as well? You are darn right it would! By helping one another we can all rise up together without waiting another day. This epitomizes the idea of the SuperHuman life.

Chapter 30

Passion to Prosperity

Prosperity is a concept that requires you to expand your mind to new possibilities. I have heard prosperity described as an ocean. If you think about the ocean as an abundant source of water, you could go to the ocean every day with a spoon and take some or you could go to the ocean every day with 1,000 dump trucks and fill them all. Either way the ocean would never go down an inch. This is the way you should think about prosperity. It is an abundant ocean of whatever you desire to achieve.

The beauty is that whatever you are passionate about is where I want you put your focus. If you are truly passionate about something it is hard to get enough of it. I want you to look at prosperity as it specifically relates to what you have passion for. That gives you the freedom to know that your prosperity is yours alone. This is the essence of passion. When you follow your passion, you are happy, filled with energy and in your heart you believe it is naturally right. Also realize that you might have passion for more than one thing. In fact it might be many things.

I wanted to be a chiropractor and I wanted to write a book. I like being an entrepreneur with everything at stake riding on my shoulders, knowing that only I will determine if I make it or break it. I know for sure that not everybody wants that, but using the tools in this book will help you find what you want or further develop your current passion.

A major part of prosperity is finances. People sometimes get a little bit weird or uncomfortable when it comes to talking about money. What I want you to understand right now is that to live in the world today you absolutely must have money. It is absolutely okay to talk about it. It is absolutely okay to want it because you do need to have it. I absolutely encourage you to go out there and earn an extremely prosperous living for yourself, and become a self-made millionaire if you desire that. Even your most basic physical needs like food, clothing and shelter require you to have enough money to pay for them. How nice these things are or how expensive they are doesn't really matter for our purposes here. What you want is going to be completely different from what someone else wants. I believe that the wrong question is "what things can my money get me?" For SuperHuman purposes, we want to look at money not necessarily in terms of what money can get you, but in terms of freedom and contribution. A better question is, "How will money free me to contribute to the world?" Therefore, you never have to worry about competing with anybody else for how much you can prosper in life.

Building prosperity in terms of financial wealth is all about using your passion and pooling your resources. It is not about throwing a bunch of investments out there to see if one pays off. Nor is it following a tip from a friend of a friend that could make you rich. I've done that and lost money because I had no passion for what I was doing. What I was really doing was gambling. That is sad because I didn't even get to enjoy the money I lost. I would have been better off spending it on gifts for others and enjoying all the happiness I was able to bring.

Your passion will guide you exactly to where you should be putting and making your money. It will also guide you to the necessary resources required to further pursue your passion. If you are passionate about real estate and property then focus on that and get good at it. If your passion is trading stocks then focus on that and take the time to become the very best at it. If your passion is business put your focus into running a successful business. If your passion is cooking do not put your focus in mutual funds. If your focus is farming organic food, then do not put your focus on stock market activity. Got it?

Live SuperHuman Tool: **Passion and resourcefulness are your biggest assets for making money.**

Your chances of winning are so much better if you focus on your passion and ways to prosper that are related to your passion. For example, you may be passionate about the stock market and even have developed some skill and made money buying and selling stocks. Instead of trying to make money in the unrelated area of rental property, you are better learning a related skill like long term investing, day trading or options trading in the stock market. Let your passion be your guide.

Major lessons can be learned about finances by making expensive mistakes. You don't have to be one of these people. Get some guidance and coaching about what to do with your money. Traditional financial planners can give you some of the worst advice if they are not experts in who you are and what your passion is.

Garrett Gunderson, financial expert and best-selling author of Killing Sacred Cows, teaches that personal finances are just that—personal. Knowing that your personal talents and passion will determine where your wealth should come from make Mr. Gunderson and his team a great SuperHuman Tool for prosperity. Old fashioned financial thinking in our current economic age could become what I call cash black holes for your money. A cash black hole is an investment that keeps your money locked away from you and does not create cash flow you can use and enjoy. New times require better strategies to keep up with a rapidly changing world of finance. SuperHumans want money they can use and enjoy during their lives. If you are saving and saving and investing to build wealth just to do so until your end, why are you doing that?

Some of the sacred cows that get killed are:

- A 401(k) is not the "safe" and "smart" **retirement** plan that you have been told it is; in fact, it's an extremely risky investment for most people.*

*I feel a 401K is an extremeley **smart savings** vehicle but **not** for retirement. Use a 401K to build up a large savings with the funds "match." Plan on paying the 10% penalty and taking the money out before retirement.

- Programs to teach you how to create safer investments that are collateralized, cash-flowing, controllable, and aligned with your expertise, passion and purpose.
- Net worth is a poor indicator of wealth and your ability to retire well.
- The proper definition of debt and how this understanding can immediately increase your prosperity.
- "High risk equals high returns" is dangerous dogma.

Finances have such an impact on you that it isn't smart or safe to leave your money in the hands of people who believe that you should do what everyone else has always done. That may not be the right thing for you. A good rule of thumb: if you don't invest your passion in it, then don't invest your money in it.

Living a SuperHuman life is a commitment to being able to help yourself, others and the world rise up to become more. Your finances are an enormous part of making that life possible. Go to LiveSuperHuman.com to help find ways to start funding your passion.

By simply reading this book as you are right now, you increase your SuperHuman capacity and your ability to be more free to feed your passion. The beauty is that becoming SuperHuman means you are expanding your mind, creativity and ability to make more money. It also can work the other way around. Making more money will increase your passion and allow you to become more SuperHuman. Be careful though, it is possible to get stuck in the rut of focusing on making money. Money isn't the only goal, living SuperHuman by focusing on what you love is. Money is the side effect of your passion. Remember first and foremost that who you are determines where you go, not the other way around.

Live SuperHuman Tool: **Who you are will determine where you go, what you create and how you will contribute. A little Zen wisdom: Be before you do.**

Here are some examples of how people's passion allowed them to be more financially free. Any one of these things could be duplicated by you if you have passion enough about the idea.

Example #1 If you are passionate about online sales:

Sell Goods Online

One of the easiest ways to do this is with eBay. I have a friend who amazes me with his ability to pick up a few hundred dollars here and there through eBay and his strategy is so simple. A couple of times a month he will stop in to a few different pawnshops to see if they have any guitars for sale. He has learned to find what he's looking for and pick it up for the right price usually $100-$400. Then he puts it on eBay and auctions it off for $600, $700 or $800. You would only have to do this once or twice a month to generate an extra $500 each and every month. This is not difficult. You just have to be a little creative and choose to specialize in one little area. You don't have to master many different trades or become expert in a number of different fields, just simply open your mind to something that might give you an opportunity you hadn't thought of before.

I have to say that this is the type of thing that anyone can do, whether they have excellent computer skills or not. Or whether they have sold anything on the Internet before or not. These websites are designed to help the inexperienced individual through the process.

Also, shop on eBay! This is an excellent way to save money. My wife has gotten Halloween costumes on eBay for 99 cents with free shipping and a free gift included! How can you beat that? Check eBay and websites like it, when you need something, you never know what kind of a deal you might find.

Example #2 If you are passionate about technology and software:

1001 Ringtones iPhone App

I have another friend who used his computer knowledge and contacts to create an iPhone application called 1001 Ring Tones. What is amazing is that it cost him nothing to get started. He simply contacted a friend who was a programmer, told him about his idea and asked if he would write the code for the program and make it work. In exchange, programmer would be paid a percentage of the sales. After the application was created and after many hours of sorting, sifting and quality checking different sounds that would become ringtones, the application was released and eventually spent serveral months in the top 10 most popular apps in the world. This application is extremely fun and still popular and generates hundreds to thousands of dollars every day in income. What a story. Now that is a SuperHuman idea!

Example #3 If you are passionate about cooking and health:

Fit Wrapz

Another example of creating your own prosperity is a friend of mine, Shigetada Toyoguchi—or Shige as I call him, has the big dream of helping people become more healthy and fit. I love that dream! His life is dedicated to this mission. Let me explain how he got there. This is a journey that I believe anyone can follow and model.

Shige started out like so many other people. He was deciding what direction he wanted to go in his schooling, working jobs such as at retail stores and the like. Eventually his interest in fitness led Shige to find his way into getting a job as a personal trainer at a local gym. To his amazement people all had the same excuses for letting their health and fitness deteriorate and came to him for help. Based on a short questionnaire he realized that nearly all his clients said they had trouble knowing the right foods to eat, choosing the right foods, cooking that food and getting time to do all that conveniently. After hearing this over and over it became clear to him that he had to find a solution to help these people. One day he asked the question to one of his clients, "If I had a balanced, healthy, pre-prepared meal for you, like a burrito of some type, would that be helpful to you?" Immediately his client was asking him where she could get them and if he had any available right then she could buy.

This is when the light bulb of bright ideas went on…ding! SuperHumans listen closely. When opportunity knocks on your door, answer it. If you have spoken to people about a topic and you continually hear of a need that people want to have filled, think about all the other people in the world who have the same need. My friend figured out that people need a new type of—for lack of a better term—fast food, or food that is healthy, balanced, customized, and less expensive but with better service to meet your schedule needs.

Shige's new company, Fit Wrapz, is dedicated to this mission by providing great tasting, wonderfully balanced, low calorie, low fat, high energy producing meals. These meals, in the form of a wrap, are perfect for today's lifestyle filled with the need for powerful food on the go. The days of fast food in the form of unhealthy meals full of large amounts of energy draining fat calories are over for SuperHumans. I want you to meet the new type of fast super food! These new foods are engineered to not only provide you with the nutrition you need, but to do it in a way that provides you better service at a lower cost than ever before. Imagine, instead of spending $5 to $8 for a fatty, processed meal you could have a healthy, balanced, fabulous tasting wrap sitting right next to you and all you have to do is reach for it.

Fast food is no longer convenient for the SuperHuman lifestyle unless it fits this guideline:

1. Balanced for your specific meal demands.
2. More cost effective.
3. More convenient.
4. Provides you with more powerful energy enhancing nutrition.
5. Tastes amazing.

I am so dedicated to making sure that we do our part to raise humanity up and away from unhealthy lifestyles, that I consider it a responsibility and moral obligation. I have committed to making sure a contribution from every purchase made at LiveSuperHuman.com (including Fit Wrapz!!!) goes to select organizations that help the world become a better place. I challenge and encourage you to team up with our rapidly growing global community of leaders, the SuperHumans, and commit yourself to this higher standard for humanity.

Stay with me because next is the last example and it's a great true story!

Example #4 If you are passionate about the stock market:

Scott's dream of prosperity had been with him for many years, but only recently did his dream lead to a tool. Scott worked in the financial services industry for more than 25 years and was acutely aware of the general lack of financial education and knowledge among the typical American family. His vision of helping others with their financial affairs led him to a variety of traditional jobs in the insurance and securities industry, and he became affiliated with large, respected financial companies. However, this traditional career path failed to match his vision. He always knew that there must be a better way, and for years he silently tinkered with innovative investment ideas and concepts, none of which were received warmly by his employers.

While Scott was vacationing in Hawaii in 2007, he noticed an advertisement for a free seminar about stock market trading taking place across the street from his hotel. You should know by now that nothing happens by accident, and in all likelihood very few people would interrupt a tropical vacation for this sort of activity. But something inside spoke to Scott and he attended the seminar. What he didn't know was that this unplanned event would eventfully develop into the biggest business venture of his life.

With only a few tips that he picked up at the seminar, Scott began reading everything he could find about stock market trading. He developed a unique trading strategy and began testing it with small amounts of money. After several months of fine tuning, Scott began to earn significant monthly profits in the stock market. Within five months he was consistently earning over $10,000 per month, with some months over $20,000, and he quit his W-2 job with a highly respected financial services firm. His friends were curious about how he was able to survive without a "job," and he shared his trading strategy with them. The friends talked to others, and one day Scott received an unsolicited request to teach his strategy, along with an offer to pay a fee for the lesson.

By the summer of 2008, Scott's "teaching" activity had evolved into a small business and Chaney Investment Strategies LLC was created. Scott's desire to guide people to a better financial life has become manifest through personal investment training, coaching and mentoring. His vision of "a better way" led him to create a self-directed investment tool that enables people to manage their own money and potentially earn 5 percent to 8 percent each and every month. Not 5 percent per year—5 percent to 8 percent per month.

Can you imagine? If you only had $50,000 to work with that could be $3,000 each month.

Nearly every SuperHuman wealth expert I've studied, such as Robert Kiyosaki best-selling author of "Rich Dad, Poor Dad," Donald Trump and Garrett strongly recommends managing your own money and not giving that control to someone else. Chaney Investment Strategies LLC helps individual investors do just that. Scott has even written an eBook that explains what he does in great detail. If managing your own money, working less and "trading for a living" is your passion or even peaks your curiosity, then I invite you to look into it.

Live SuperHuman Tool: **End tolerance! Don't allow yourself to settle for tolerating anything less than your passion. In order to Live SuperHuman you want to treat YOU like the precious gift you are. This means making the world around you better for yourself. Don't tolerate wasteful living from yourself or those around you. This doesn't mean don't ever have a hamburger if you want one or don't buy an expensive car if you want and can easily do so. You absolutely should do these things now and then. Just don't tolerate living your life ignorant to the continuous decay around you. Take action toward your passion!**

This is an example of how customizing what you want out of life and what you see as personal prosperity can be created for you. Maybe you don't want to create a business and be an entrepreneur. Maybe you just want to make your money work for you so that you can be free from having to think about working at a job and taking time away from your family. Maybe you want to move to a tropical island and open snow cone shack. Maybe you always wanted to sing the national anthem at a baseball game. Or maybe you always wanted to open a bird shelter. It really doesn't matter what the thing is, just remember that the thing is your thing! Just knowing what that thing is gives you SuperHuman powers, dreams, goals, hope, and the ability to make it happen.

Chapter 31

Cleaning House

I have heard it said that the three of the most difficult things to do in communication are:

1. To give love in response to hate.
2. To defend someone who is not present to defend themselves.
3. To admit when you are wrong.

I'd agree that those things are all very difficult, however, I believe that there is something that is more difficult than those listed above. I believe the hardest thing in life is not to become desensitized to your surroundings. It is part of human nature to adapt. We even discussed earlier that the most important job of the nervous system is adaptation, which is healthy and necessary. However, I feel that in many situations one can forget to be grateful for what they have, always wanting the next best thing. Beware, and rise above this desire by connecting to the feelings of how excited you were when things were new.

There are many ways to illustrate the desensitization phenomenon and you see it over and over again in the world and in your own life. People who became wealthy from nothing can forget how hard it was when they had little money. People in relationships who used to get turned on by their partner may stop being stimulated as much, yet the partner is just as wonderful/sexy as they used to be. You see it all the time in situations in which people are unhappy with their current life situation even though they have more to be grateful for than most other people on the planet.

There are many ways this can happen or be described, but usually it is something that sneaks up on you. It is like gaining 1 pound per year for 30 years and then all of a sudden you look down say, "How did I get to be 30 pounds over weight?" Do everything you can not to let this happen.

If this happens to you and you have a realization that you have been taking things for granted or desensitized to something in your life, here is what I recommend you do before you react:

1. Determine if this thing/situation is something you still want. This step should be easy. Yes, I want to lose weight. Yes, I love my spouse and want them in my life. No, I don't need that constant-source-of-negativity friend or relative anymore.

2. Determine if this thing/situation is still related to your purpose. This step can be more challenging because your purpose can change over time. This may be a good time to re-evaluate your purpose. This can also be hard emotionally. You may find that this thing/situation is a result of living off purpose or with no purpose at all. This is a bad sign. Use this as an opportunity to get back on course quickly!

3. Take action and find a solution now! Typically, if you find you want to keep this thing/situation then the solution will be related to gratitude. You will want to stir up deep gratitude for the thing/situation. Get back to the experience of how much you appreciated it when it was new. If you no longer want the thing/situation then get rid of it or cut off contact with it or get counseling or trusted advice to help you move on.

Chapter 32

You Matter

You will find that, literally, the content of many books, magazines and sources contain the exact opposite of what is talked about and recommended in this book, which is truly aimed at pulling you out of the old ways of living and launching you into a new way of thinking, acting and treating yourself.

I love each and every one of you for being open-minded, for searching for something new, for wanting to expand yourself, for wanting to help others, and for wanting to make a difference. I know in my heart—and I can virtually guarantee—that if you apply the tools and tips laid out for you here in this book your life will change for the better. I believe that when your life changes for the better, other people will notice and you will be able to help others change their lives for the better with an authority and confidence you never dreamed of having before.

Right now I'm going to ask you to do something that will take you 10 or 15 minutes. You have come this far, the next step may be your most important one. I want you to get a pen or pencil. After finishing the next page, I want you to tear out page 137 with the blank lines on it. And I want you to go back through the book and make a list of the things in this book that you thought would make a difference in your life in only one or two words each. I'm talking about the things that stood out to you when you read them and you thought something like "I should do that" or "I want to do that and I know I can." It could be a simple tip, a Live SuperHuman Tool, or a piece of advice you that you should share with someone. Start now before you read the next paragraph and write down a minimum of five but no more than 10 items. Ready, go...

Great work, I'm excited for you and thank you! Now I want you to circle only two of the points you just wrote down. Find just one thing that you are going to implement right now at this very moment. If one of them was do yoga then put the book down and do some yoga now. If one of them was call a friend and tell them about what you read then put the book down and do it now. It doesn't matter what time it is! If one of them was to get yourself some better supplements then put the book down and get on the computer and order some supplements. If one of them was to do some meditation then put the book down and go sit comfortably and meditate. Whatever it is, take the action now. You will find it is much easier than you think and you will feel so good about yourself for actually doing it right now. Trust me, I have been there, I have done this and I know that you will build your self-esteem if you do it now.

Some of the best advice I've ever heard, which really isn't advice at all, it is truth, comes from Dr. Nathaniel Branden who is a recognized by psychologists as the world's leading authority on self-esteem. I have heard him say, "Your life matters."

I tell you this so that you live everyday from now on knowing that:

Your safety matters.
Your love matters.
Your health matters.
Your happiness matters.
Your prosperity matters.
Your life matters.

From now on, in everything that you do, **know without doubt that you matter** and this is the essence of the quest to Live SuperHuman.

Live SuperHuman Tool Summary

All the tools in one place, right where you need them!

Chapter 3

- Thinking bigger and more creatively is a way to charge up and become more powerful.

- Gratitude builds your power.

- Yoga will make you physically and Neuro-Spiritually more powerful.

- Meditate to increase wellness, Physically and Neuro-Spiritually.

Chapter 4

- Share positive energy with everyone you know in the form of a blessing. You never know who may need it right now.

Chapter 5

- A SuperHuman power that will help us all is the power to be present, to live and focus on what is happening now without fearfully worrying about the future or living with constant guilt over the past. When you feel guilt, you are living in the past. When you feel fear, you are living in the future. Your super powers come from being present! All your strength is generated by focusing on what you are doing right here, right now.

Chapter 6

- A child becomes SuperHuman if the parent does three things instead of giving externally focused praise: says what they see, notices effort rather than offering external praise, and asks children how they feel about their accomplishments in a declaratory manner.

Chapter 8

- Always be honest with yourself and with others.

- The two best tools to help free your body from the negative effects of emotional stress are chiropractic care and questioning your thoughts about anything that causes you negative stress.

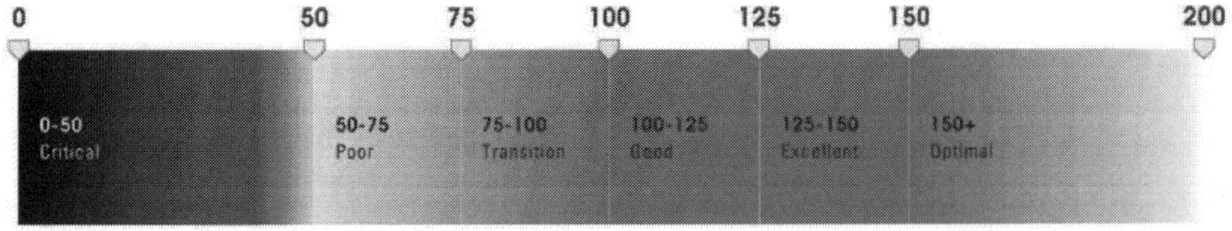

Chapter 9

- The 5 Blessings are a legitimate, simple and powerful way you can consistently enhance your well being. Use these tools as described to raise your own wellness and those around you.

Chapter 10

- Use this scale to identify your level of wellness right now. Pick a spot on the scale where you think you are and circle it. Zero represents ill health or death and 200 is the most optimal level of wellness you can imagine for yourself. What matters is not where actually are, but where you think you are on the scale. And no matter where you actually are, you can always do better. The SuperHuman Elements of Wellness will help move you to higher levels of well being. Read on!

Chapter 11

- Chiropractors are the only doctors who correct subluxations, or nerve disturbance, restoring proper communication in the central nervous system. Healthy nerve communication will then produce healthier function in your organs, cells and systems.

- Build muscle strength 3 different ways to help lose weight!

Chapter 12

- Strengthen flexibility to ease suffering with pain and tell everyone know how you felt better through increased flexibility. Use the resources in this chapter to implement LS code principles 2 (always share your powers with as many people as possible) and 3 (always help others, and the world, whenever you can)!

- Use the Accelerated Recovery Performance Trainer to help heal injuries and eliminate pain.

- Use the SuperStretch Towel program to get and stay super fit.

- SuperHumans don't hesitate, they act! Before now, many opportunities to improve your life have been ignored. Just like super heroes act quickly to save someone's life, it is even more important SuperHumans act quickly to save their own lives! If you don't save your own life now, you will be no good to anybody else later.

Chapter 14

- Develop consistency by finding one small change that you have wanted to make. Do not pick something hard. Instead, pick something very easy, something that amounts to a 3 percent change rather than a 25 percent change or 50 percent change. For example let's say you have wanted to get up earlier every morning by about 30 minutes so you can have extra time to do any number of healthier things like exercise, eat a better breakfast, or just have more time to spend with your family. Instead of setting your alarm for 30 minutes earlier tomorrow, go to your clock right now and set your alarm for two or three minutes earlier. Then allow yourself to get up three minutes earlier every day for a week. After a week, set your alarm for 3 to 5 minutes earlier again and do the same thing for a week. You can use this 3 percent change method in every aspect of your life in which you want something to be different.

Chapter 14

- To lose weight you must burn more calories than you consume. Period. The healthier the calories, the healthier and lighter you will be! You are what you eat as they say … so don't eat junk! You are too good for that. Treat your body as a temple, a spiritual place where only good things are allowed in.

Chapter 15

- Nutritional Typing is recognized as one of the very best ways to eat your food. Find out your Nutritional Type today!

Chapter 17

- Expand your GAP with powerful supplements and regular chiropractic care to remove subluxations.

Chapter 18

- Stay away from milk that is not 100 percent organic and raw. Sheep milk is best, then goat, and finally cow milk. Very few states allow raw milk to be produced and sold legally. Alternatives are rice and soy. Recent studies advise avoiding soy consumption in large amounts because it has estrogen hormone mimicking properties. Rice, however, does not have high nutrient value but is inexpensive and usually organic.

Chapter 19

- Science estimates the human body averages over 10,000 potential opportunities to develop cancer per day! Lowering your risk of cancer is a superpower you naturally have by being strong and healthy. Strengthen this power through improving Bio-chemical & Neuro-spiritual health.

Chapter 22

- A major cause of heart attacks is the fact that when cholesterol is oxidized it builds up in your arteries faster. Prevent heart attacks with nutritional supplements designed to prevent oxidation. Reduce total cholesterol levels in your blood by following other SuperHuman lifestyle tips recommended in this book.

- SuperHumans know they have the power to help save others. They never doubt this power and act decisively to share it with others. I believe that I can help you learn how to do exactly that. Share the information with others, so that you, too, can help save others.

Chapter 23

- Fighting diseases is a superpower! Take multiple kinds of top quality antioxidants and the best multi vitamins to strengthen your disease fighting super powers.

Chapter 25

- Do everything you can to avoid getting a flu shot.

Chapter 26

- Break the mold. You are not an everyday citizen, you are a super citizen who knows that knowledge is one of your Super Powers. Educate yourself on the risks and benefits of any treatment (or anything at all), before you allow yourself or your family to receive it. Make an informed decision; don't just do what everyone else does.

Chapter 30

- Passion and resourcefulness are your biggest assets for making money.

- Who you are will determine where you go, what you create and how you will contribute. A little Zen wisdom: Be before you do.

- End tolerance! Don't allow yourself to settle for tolerating anything less than your passion. In order to Live SuperHuman you want to treat YOU like the precious gift you are. This means making the world around you better for yourself. Don't tolerate wasteful living from yourself or those around you. This doesn't mean don't ever have a hamburger if you want one or don't buy an expensive car if you want and can easily do so. You absolutely should do these things now and then. Just don't tolerate living your life ignorant to the continuous decay around you. Take action toward your passion!

Live SuperHuman Sources

1. Radin D, Lund N, Emoto M, Kizu T: Effects of Distant Intention on Water Crystal Formation: A Triple-Blind Replication. Journal of Scientific Exploration 2008;22(8):481

2. Web-MD, http://www.webmd.com/sex-relationships/features/10-surprising-health-benefits-of-sex.

3. http://www.lef.org/magazine/mag2006/aug2006_report_death_01.htm

4. Fowler JA, Christakis NA: Dynamic spread of happiness in a large social network: longitudinal analysis over 20 years in the Framingham Heart Study. BMJ 2008;337:a2338.

5. http://www.webmd.com/diet/news/20030827/dark-chocolate-is-healthy-chocolate.

6. Samuel S. Epstein, MD: Aug. 29, 2006 press release titled "Hormonal Milk Poses Greater Risks Than Just Twinning," to support his book What's In Your Milk?

7. Martin Donohoe, MD, and Rick North: August 31, 2006 article "Errors in MSNBC Story on Organic Milk."

8. Enhancement of chemotherapy by manipulation of tumour pH. Raghunand N, He X, van Sluis R, Mahoney B, Baggett B, Taylor CW, Paine-Murrieta G, Roe D, Bhujwalla ZM, Gillies RJ. Arizona Cancer Center.

9. Weinstein RA. Nosocomial Infection Update. Special Issue. Emerging Infectious Diseases. Vol 4 No. 3, July Sept 1998.

10. www.health-report.co.uk/prescription_drugs_kill.html.

11. Pattison N, Warren L. 2002 drug industry profits: hefty pharmaceutical company margins dwarf other industries. Washington (DC): Public Citizen Congress Watch; June 2003. Available: www.citizen.org/documents/Pharma_Report.pdf

12. Philip Day, "Cancer: Why we're still dying to know the truth", Credence Publications, 2000

13. www.abcnews.go.com/Health/ColdandFluNews/story?id=6418974&page=1

14. Forbes.com 2006

15. Circulation 1992, British Medical Journal 1996, Journal of the American Medical Association 1997

16. Peet M, Brind J, Ramchand CN, Shah S, Vankar GK (2001). "Two double-blind placebo-controlled pilot studies of eicosapentaenoic acid in the treatment of schizophrenia". Schizophrenia Research 49 (3): 243–51. doi:0.1016/S0920-9964(00)00083-9. PMID 11356585. http://jerrycott.com/user/peet.pdf

17. Song C, Zhao S (Oct 2007). "Omega-3 fatty acid eicosapentaenoic acid. A new treatment for psychiatric and neurodegenerative diseases: a review of clinical investigations". Expert Opin Investig Drugs 16 (10): 1627–38. doi:10.1517/13543784.16.10.1627. PMID 17922626

18. Huan M, Hamazaki K, Sun Y, Itomura M, Liu H, Kang W, Watanabe S, Terasawa K, Hamazaki T. (2004). "Suicide attempt and n-3 fatty acid levels in red blood cells: a case control study in China" (abstract). Biological psychiatry 56 (7): 490–6. doi:10.1016/j.biopsych.2004.06.028. PMID 1540784

19. www.journals.elsevierhealth.com/periodicals/bps/article/PIIS0006322304007061/abstract

20. Hardman,W Elaine. (n-3) Fatty Acids and Cancer Therapy. http://jn.nutrition.org/cgi/content/full/134/12/3427S.

21. Fernandez, Esteve; Liliane Chatenoud, Carlo La Vecchia, Eva Negri, and Silvia Franceschi (1999). "Fish consumption and cancer risk". http://www.thedcasite.com/Omega3_Fatty_acids/Fish_consumption_and_cancer_risk.pdf. Retrieved 2009-10-05

22. Meharban Singh (March 2005). "Essential Fatty Acids, DHA and the Human Brain from the Indian Journal of Pediatrics, Volume 72" (PDF).

23. medind.nic.in/icb/t05/i3/icbt05i3p239.pdf. Retrieved October 8, 2007. doi:10.1016/j.prostaglandins.2004.03.005. PMID 15290791.

24. McNamara RK, Hahn CG, Jandacek R, et al. (2007). "Selective deficits in the omega-3 fatty acid docosahexaenoic acid in the postmortem orbitofrontal cortex of patients with major depressive disorder". Biol. Psychiatry 62 (1): 17–24. doi:10.1016/j.biopsych.2006.08.026. PMID 17188654.

25. "DHA Deficit Detected in Frontal Cortex of Severely Depressed Patients". Fats of Life. September 2007. http://fatsoflife.com/pufa/article.asp?nid=1&edition=this&id=493. Retrieved 2007-10-31.

26. Schønberg SA, Lundemo AG, Fladvad T, Holmgren K, Bremseth H, Nilsen A, Gederaas O, Tvedt KE, Egeberg KW, Krokan HE (2006). "Closely related colon cancer cell lines display different sensitivity to polyunsaturated fatty acids, accumulate different lipid classes and downregulate sterol regulatory element-binding protein 1". Cancer Lett. 273 (12): 2749–65. PMID 16817902.

27. Shaikh IAA, Brown I, Schofield AC, Wahle KWJ, Heys SD (November 2008). "Docosahexaenoic acid enhances the efficacy of docetaxel in prostate cancer cells by modulation of apoptosis: the role of genes associated with the NF-kappaB pathway." Prostate. 68 (15): 1635–1646. doi:10.1002/pros.20830. PMID 18668525.

28. http://www.webmd.com/cold-and-flu/news/20040115/flu-vaccine-missed-its-mark-this-year, http://blogs.wsj.com/health/2008/02/13/this-seasons-flu-vaccine-misses-many-marks

29. http://www.cdc.gov/flu/about/qa/season.htm

30. Jefferson T, Di Piertrantonj C, Rivetti A, Bawazeer GA, At-Ansary LA, Ferroni E: Vaccines for preventing influenza in healthy adults. Cochrane Database Syst Rev 2010 Jul 7;(7);CD001269.

31. www.spontaneouscreation.org/SC/VaccineOffer.htm

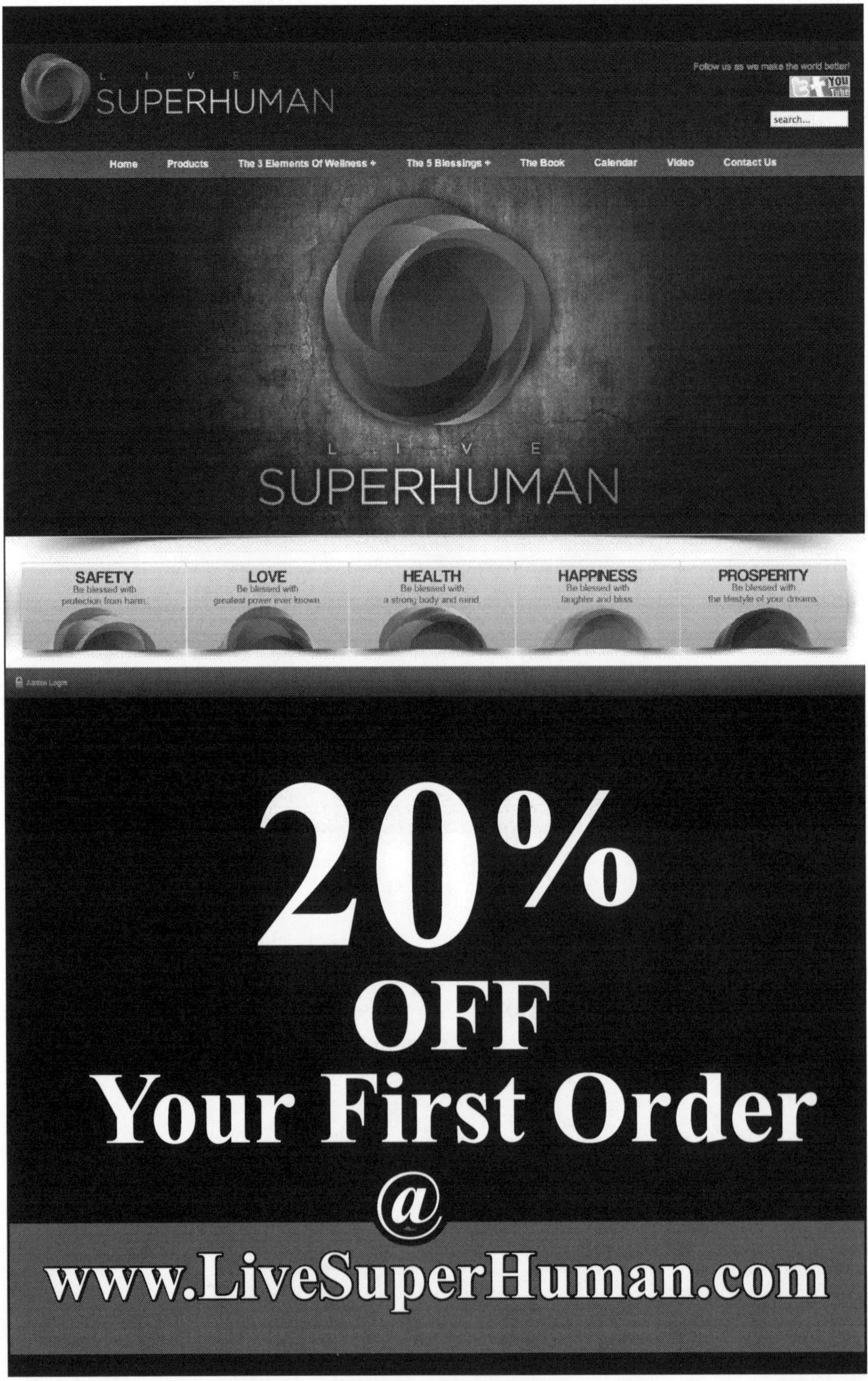
L I V E
SUPERHUMAN
Follow us as we make the world better!
search...
Home
Products
The 3 Elements Of Wellness +
The 5 Blessings +
The Book
Calendar
Video
Contact Us
L I V E
SUPERHUMAN
SAFETY
Be blessed with
protection from harm.
LOVE
Be blessed with
greatest power ever known.
HEALTH
Be blessed with
a strong body and mind.
HAPPINESS
Be blessed with
laughter and bliss.
PROSPERITY
Be blessed with
the lifestyle of your dreams.

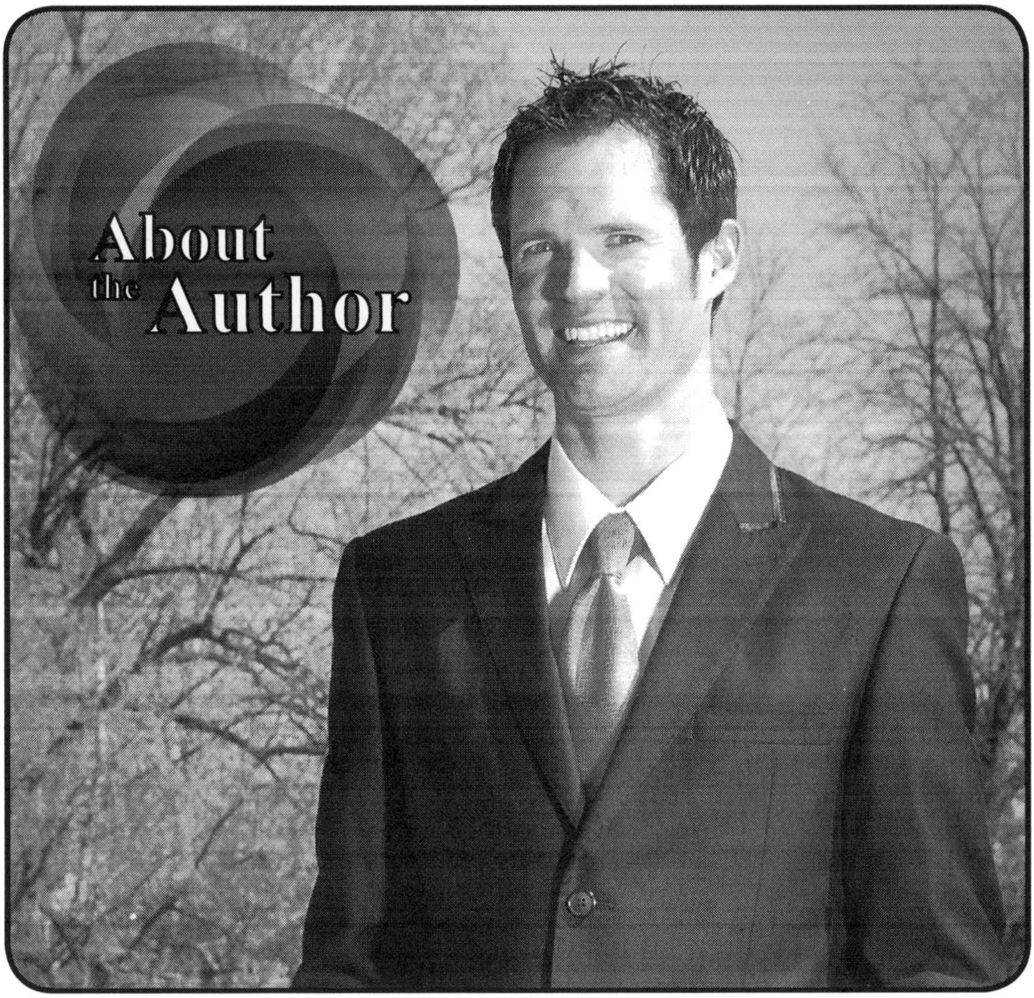

Dr. Rook Torres earned the degrees of Doctor of Chiropractic and Bachelor of Science in Nutrition by the age of 23. Dr. Torres' entrepreneurial spirit led to his first lawn care business at the age of 12, and currently, he runs his own family wellness practice he opened over decade ago. The Live SuperHuman book and brand is the realization of an undying passion to see people become more healthy, self-confident, successful, safe, loved and loving. Dr. Torres laughs as he says, "My dream is that if I can make the world a better place for others then it will naturally become a better place for me, my family and those I care about. I want you to benefit every bit as much…I urge you to make this your dream too!" Dr. Torres has taught in hospitals, authored dozens of original lectures, and treated tens of thousands of office visits. He stays on the cutting edge of current scientific research, healthcare philosophy and politics. There is no more qualified and caring authority to bring this information to you.

17748096R00102

Made in the USA
Lexington, KY
25 September 2012